WATER ROULETTE

WATER ROULETTE

BILL STRAIT

Dedicated to my loving family, Anna, Brittany, and Perry.

Table of Contents

Foreword

I thought I knew water. After all, I drink it every day. We don't usually think much about it here in America, we just consume it, bathe in it, boil it, make ice out of it, mix it with Irish whiskey, or do any one of hundreds of other things with it. Sadly, such is not the case in most parts of the world, and I have learned through this book that it may not be the case in America for very long.

What I also learned was that the water I thought I was drinking isn't really the water that I am actually consuming, and that we have been lulled into what is frequently a false comfort zone when it comes to our water.

I have also learned that Bill Strait is a man of great knowledge and great vision. What Bill has seen up close has given him insight that is truly a treasure. Few people in the world can say that they have literally been around the world hundreds of times. During these many years of travel he has seen and studied water conditions in more countries than I can name and many more countries than I can spell. Bill's breadth of experience is unequaled in this arena. When he talks about water, I listen closely.

This book is enlightening, and sometimes frightening. There is information here that every American needs to know, and that every citizen of the world should not overlook. Water Roulette is an uncommon book, and hopefully will convert many people into water activists.

Bob Hackney

Lawyer, Author, and water lover.

- Lawyer's Guide to Blockchain Technology: What it is and how it will disrupt the practice of law
- Entrepreneur's Guide to the New Equity Crowdfunding Rules: Business Law Series
- Let's Bring America Back
- Mergers & Acquisitions 101
  (Available on Amazon.com)

March 15, 2017

Introduction

I started my aviation career flying seaplanes in the Louisiana Delta. Taking off and landing on the mighty Mississippi River, beautiful bayous, and canals was a constant reminder of all things water. I went on to spend 35 years circumnavigating the earth during my airline-captain career for a world-wide company, retiring on the trusty Boeing 747.

My pilot travels around the world were progressively disturbed by vague notions that the water in those 40+ countries of my travels may not have been safe to drink, gargle with, or bathe in. Those trips included over 300 ocean crossings and provided me an opportunity to observe massive amounts of ocean water that appeared to be readily available for use. My 260 trips around the earth also provided a front row seat to raging rivers, tranquil lakes, and pristine ponds.

It is difficult for us to imagine any scarcity of clean water-at-large, drinking water in particular. Water toxicity and occasional droughts here in the U.S.A., however, are a fact of life in our modern era.

It was on one particular trip of many to Mumbai, from my room in a four-star hotel, that I was confronted with a view directly into a slum. I later learned that it was unaffectionate called "visqueen city," a sad reference to the plastic roofing there. The conspicuously dirty water flowing through the slum made it obvious that whatever was coming out of the faucet in my room was also going to be unclean. This suspicion was confirmed when drawing a bath in the hotel offered up a tub of brownish liquid. The idle thoughts that had been lurking in my mind regrading water purity came into sharp focus during that particular sojourn.

In that hotel room, I observed the complimentary bottled water bore a label that was vague at best as to the exact contents … was it water or something else? Whatever it was, it had obviously originated within the city below. It was an epiphany of sorts and put me in mind of a classic *Saturday Night Live* commercial parody, starring Bill Murray, as he lifted a bottle of obviously filthy water and said "Swill: everything you always wanted in a mineral water, and more."

In my much earlier days as a kid in Harvey, Louisiana, water was usually drunk, in the memorable informality of the times, from the garden hose laying in the yard. No thought was given to the purity, sanctity, or safety of that H_2 and O, as youthful playing was the order of those light-hearted days.

In those years, no particular water caution or environmental concern appeared to be in effect as my Dad and I headed by bus to the Audubon Park municipal pool for our weekly swimming trips. The water would be cool, and a fun time was assured! Looking back, the pool authorities had taken the precaution of requiring a shower beforehand (often faked with a few lazy splashes) and having us step in a little trough of foul, pine-oil smelling liquid, before running for the water. Those were my carefree days, long before I made a good living flying seaplanes on the water.

For years, America has been spared the water quality and quantity issues that have plagued most other countries. That is changing dramatically as we speak. We are all headed for a reckoning in the game of Water Roulette.

On that particular trip to India I was transformed from being merely water curious. I became a card carrying water-world concerned citizen! It should begin to concern us all as we start recognizing our dependence on H_2O. After all, scientists advise that we humans, our pets, and livestock will actually die without water in three to five days! We have enough worries. We shouldn't have to be preoccupied with the sanctity, availability, and purity of water, even if we have taken it for granted all our lives!

I made the decision then and there to research the subject of water: it became my avocation, and then my passion. I have spent virtually all of my spare time over many years, and countless miles of travel, researching issues of drinking water purity and scarcity.

There are many problems in our drinking water today, both in quality and quantity. There are many solutions, many of which are not obvious. Each approach to solving our drinking water conundrum comes with a cost: to us the consumers, our society, and our political landscape.

The objective of this book is to finally separate fact from fantasy and discover the truth regarding drinking water impurities and scarcity, and to raise public awareness of the advancing, multi-layered problems that most of the world faces daily — and that we Americas face now and in the near future. We will also explore some ways to improve and manage our personal fortunes in the water casino.

I may exercise literary license and touch on a few conspiracy theories, and use metaphors, typos, and perhaps humor in the process!

Nothing here is intended as health advice. I am not a medical practitioner of any sort, and I do not play one on television. I am, however, a student of all things water, and welcome all open and honest discussions, illuminations, and refinements on the subject.

The first step is understanding. Let's set sail into dark waters, and hope that, by gaining a better understanding of the issues, we can all participate in solutions. Come sail away with me!

Chapter

1

WATER UP CLOSE, WATER IS US

THE PHYSICALITY OF WATER

What is water, really? Two atoms of hydrogen and one atom of oxygen equals water. Water is a molecule: it is made from atoms that have been chemically combined. It is also a compound because the atoms that make up water are not all the same. That's it, class dismissed. In the modern era there have been many attempts to romanticize this elementary fact.

What is in our drinking water besides hydrogen and oxygen? That is really the critical question.

Water is heavy, at 8.345404 pounds per gallon. It is incompressible, and expensive to transport, by way of a reported 1,000,000 miles of pipe and pumps, or via handy bottles. In the U.S.A., 3.9 trillion gallons are consumed from the tap in one month, at an average cost of $0.002, or two-tenths of a cent, per gallon. A trillion anything is a lot, as we shall examine later.

Dr. Gerald Pollack is Founding Editor-in-Chief of the scientific journal *WATER*, and is recognized worldwide as a one of the leader and premier research scientists in the water physics. In his intriguing work, *The Fourth Phase of Water: Beyond Solid, Liquid, and Vapor* (http://www.

ebneranderson.com), he reveals the secrets of the world's most common substance. Water is not always H_2O, and actually transforms itself into a so-called Exclusion-Zone (EZ), with a formula of H_3O_2, when touching most surfaces.

Dr. Pollack goes on to explain that:

- Our bodies are 99 percent water molecules, but the water in our cells is endowed with special purposes.
- The mysteriously-structured H_3O_2 is more viscous and dense, has a negative charge, and can hold and deliver energy, much like a battery.
- The key ingredient in this structured water is light, much like electromagnetic energy.
- As we spend time in the sun or in a laser sauna, we charge our cells.

A little farther out there: is consciousness and water intertwined and related to plant life? One of the original pioneers in his water consciousness studies, Dr. Marcel Vogel, determined that when bulk water was in the process of freezing, excess energy is extracted from the water. Dr. Vogel also noted that, at this juncture, water molecules develop a consciousness, "a memory, a knowing of what they were designed to do and to be."

Farther still, Dr. Masaru Emoto explains in his book, *The Hidden Messages in Water*, his startling discovery that there is molecular evidence that words and thoughts change the structure of cells in our water. Emoto was born in Yokohama, Japan and received certification from the Open International University as a Doctor of Alternative Medicine. He gained worldwide acclaim through his groundbreaking research and discovery that water is deeply connected to our individual and collective consciousness. He undertook extensive research of water around the planet and realized that it was only in the frozen crystal form that water showed us its true nature. He describes: "The idea to freeze water and observe it with a microscope came upon me. With this method, I was convinced that I should be able to see something like snow crystals."

After two months of trial and error, this idea bore fruit and beautifully shining hexagonal crystals were created from the invisible world. At first, he observed crystals of tap water, river water, and lake water. From tap water there were no beautiful crystals. They could not find any crystals from frozen water of rivers and lakes near big cities, either. However, from the water from rivers and lakes where water is kept pristine and far from development, they reportedly observe beautiful crystals, with each one unique.

The researchers exposed the water to various conditions and observed the results: showing letters to water, showing pictures to water, playing music to water, and praying over water.

"The result was that we always observed beautiful crystals after giving good words, playing good music, and offering pure prayer to water. On the other hand, when negative thoughts and emotions were focused intentionally upon the water, the water crystals displayed were chaotic, fragmented structures. Moreover, we never observed identical crystals." - *The Hidden Messages in Water* by Masaru Emoto, 2004

Drs. Pollack, Vogel, and Emoto and I would get along famously!

What's the deal? Can singing to water, having good thoughts near it, shaking it a certain way, magnetizing it, or doing any variation of these things change our most abundant and essential resource in some magical way? Water is much maligned, enshrined, politicized, and forever romanticized.

> **"They both listened silently to the water, which to them was not just water, but the voice of Being, the voice of perpetual Becoming."**
>
> - Herman Hesse, *Siddhartha*

WHERE OUR WATER ORIGINATES

Where does our drinking water originate from, creationists notwithstanding? It has to start somewhere. It is a cycle, and brilliant scientists report that water, at the molecular level, is never destroyed! That is a relief, of sorts. We'll pick up the chase with the molecules rising from the earth's surface:

The hydrologic cycle starts with evaporation from surface water of oceans. As the moisture is lifted, it cools, and the resulting vapor forms clouds from condensation. The atmosphere holds 37.5 million billion gallons of water in the invisible vapor phase. Air currents carry these clouds around the world until precipitation returns the water to the surface of the earth. From there it either evaporates again, or seeps into the ground to become groundwater. We imagine the gentle breeze as we breathe the mist deeply.

Groundwater seeps into the oceans, streams, and rivers, or is released through transpiration back into the atmosphere. The water remaining on the surface is called runoff, and it ultimately empties into the lakes, streams, and rivers, where it flows back to the oceans to begin the trip again. Kind of a circle of life.

There are two paths to the atmosphere for the mysterious water molecules: evaporation and transpiration. Evaporation, as above, is the process by which liquid water is transformed into a gaseous state. A further requirement for the process is that water is available and that the relative humidity is less than that of the evaporating surface. Transpiration is the release of water from plants into the atmosphere.

Surface water (streams, rivers, and lakes) or ground water (in the aquifer, a natural underground layer, often of sand or gravel, that contains water) can serve as sources of drinking water, referred to as source water. Source water provides water for public drinking, water supplies, and private water wells.

Where do we get our drinking water today, in the common era? Icecaps and glaciers are responsible for 68.7%, groundwater 30.1%, other 9%, and surface water 3%. It is pumped from the top eight river basins for water to Americans: from the mighty Mississippi, St. Lawrence Columbia, Nelson Brazos, San Joaquin, Sacramento and Colorado — and they all flow into the Atlantic, Pacific, and Arctic Oceans (according to www.allianceforwaterefficiency.org).

"Yes, we'll gather at the river, the beautiful, the beautiful river; Gather with the saints at the river. That flows by the throne of God."

- Robert Lowery,
1864; first published in *Happy Voices*, 1865

WATER IN OUR BODIES

How does water sustain us? A study of cellular hydration is essential to our understanding. We're going to start small by looking through the microscope at cellular microbiology. Rest assured, there will not be a final exam in chemistry or biology. It is intriguing that cell dehydration can be the root cause of many ills. We will go inside us and take a look around … kind of like the 1987 movie *Innerspace*. Dennis Quaid and Martin Short seemed to know their way around in there.

Note that we need it for naturally moisturizing our skin and to ensure proper cellular formation underneath our layers of skin. Water also regulates the temperature of the human body. It also removes wastes from us.

The experts offer advice for our water-well-being. Dr. Stephen Sinatra is a highly respected and sought-after cardiologist whose integrative approach to treating cardiovascular disease has revitalized patients with even the most advanced forms of illness. Dr. Sinatra's expertise is grounded in more than 35 years of clinical practice.

Dr. Sinatra advises us that remaining properly hydrated has a great benefit of normalizing blood pressure! He explains that not drinking enough water forces the body to attempt to retain its fluid by sodium retention. The body also closes down some of its vital capillary beds during dehydration, putting pressure on our arteries and capillaries resulting in elevated blood pressure.

Dos and Don'ts for Lowering Your Blood Pressure Naturally With Water:

DO drink the right amount of water. To get the maximum health benefits of drinking water, you need to drink eight to ten 8-ounce glasses of water per day.

DON'T overdo it. While I want you to get the health benefits of drinking water, I don't want you to go overboard. Like a sponge. your body can absorb water at a limited rate. It will require some time to adapt to your new level of water intake and become fully hydrated. Drinking too much water can overwork your kidneys and digestive system…

DO drink more water when you exercise. You lose water through sweat and evaporation. So, to get the full benefits of drinking water you want to hydrate well before, during, and after exercise… (You can learn more from Dr. Sinatra at www.drsinatra.com.)

Dr. F. Batmanghelidj was trained at St Mary's Hospital Medical, and practiced medicine in the United Kingdom before his return to his native Iran. He claimed to have discovered the medicinal value of water in treating the pain of peptic ulcers during his detention in prison, by treating inmates with water when medication was not available.

In 1992, he authored *Your Body's Many Cries for Water. Your Body's Many Cries for Water* (http://www.watercure.com). In this book, Dr. Batmanghelidj asserts that chronic dehydration is the root cause of most pain and many ailments, opposing the use of drugs to cure conditions that he claimed could instead be addressed by increased water consumption.

According to the late F. Batmanghelidj's fascinating book, the human brain, at only one fiftieth of our body weight, uses 18 to 20 percent of our blood flow! Our bodies are 60% water and our organs are composed of water: the brain is composed of 80% water; blood is 83% water; lungs, 79%; muscles, 76%. The brain sends out a host of chemical messengers in its job of water maestro.

Dr. Batmanghelidj draws a convincing association of the physiology of stress and the body's response to dehydration. Our body goes into the "fight or flight" response, then goes into action: strong hormones are secreted and remain active until the body gets out of the stressful state. What triggers the response? Perhaps stress at work, or a tiger is attacking patrons at the mall with us there. When we are dehydrated our bodies go into the "fight or flight" mode irrespective of our consciousness of it. Same body response, either dehydrated or attacked by a tiger. The brain demands additional hydration because of the stress, which keeps the "stress spiral" going:

> Endorphins prepare the body to endure hardship and injury until it is out of danger. They also raise the pain threshold...with the "umbrella" of endorphins, the body will be able to continue its task.

> Cortisone will initiate the remobilization of stored energy and raw materials. Fat is broken down into fatty acids to be converted into energy. Some proteins are once again broken down into the basic amino acids for the formation of extra neurotransmitters, new proteins, and some special amino acids to be burned by the muscles..... If the action of cortisone continues for long, soon there will be some selective depletion from the amino acid reserves of the body, thus the body continues to "feed off itself."

> Vasopressin regulates the selective flow of water into some cells of the body. It also causes a constriction of the capillaries it activates...it causes vasoconstriction. It is produced in the pituitary gland and secreted into the circulation...

> Prolactin is a protein that, in humans, is best known for enabling females to produce milk. It increases with stress, and is associated with inflammation. As we become progressively dehydrated, the stress response causes essential services to various organs to shut off because the brain is operating the switchboard.

> The operating mechanisms for adaptation to dehydration, which will climax into vasoconstriction, are the same as mentioned for stress...they close a number of open

capillaries in the vascular bed and increase the pressure in the rest to squeeze water through the membranes into the cells in 'priority organs' ...Dehydration is the number one stressor of the human body, or any living matter. (https://theinnozablog.blogspot.ca/2012/09/endorphins-cortisone-prolactin-and.html)

Dr. Batmanghelidj's successful treatment of many serious infirmities, with his inexpensive treatment regimen, challenges many foundational beliefs about health care as practiced today. Perhaps, as the good doctor suggests, the truth lies in that much of diseases, may serious in nature, result from the dehydration of various body parts therein, and perhaps much of that dehydration is imbalances in our intake of water and salt. The final exam for us to determine our personal hydration is simply to observe the color of our urine: clear is the objective. Perhaps we can find relief from our ills by following the late Doctor's controversial advice: drink water throughout the day.

"If you're well hydrated, your heart doesn't have to work as hard," said John Batson, M.D., a sports medicine physician with Lowcountry Spine & Sport in Hilton Head Island, S.C., and an American Heart Association volunteer.

Dehydration can be a serious condition that can lead to problems ranging from swollen feet or a headache to life-threatening illnesses such as heat stroke.

What does being well-hydrated mean? The amount of water a person needs depends on climatic conditions, clothing worn, and exercise intensity and duration, Batson said. A person who perspires heavily will need to drink more than someone who doesn't. Certain medical conditions, such as diabetes or heart disease, may also mean you need to drink more water. People with cystic fibrosis have high concentrations of sodium in their sweat and need to use caution to avoid dehydration. And some medications can act as diuretics, causing the body to lose more fluid.

Thirst isn't the best indicator that you need to drink. "If you get thirsty, you're already dehydrated," Batson said.

Water is best. For most people, water is the best thing to drink to stay hydrated. Sources of water also include foods, such as fruits and vegetables that contain a high percentage of water.

High Water Content Fruit:

Watermelon and strawberries contain about 92 percent water per volume. Other fruits with high water content include grapefruit with 91 percent, cantaloupe with 90 percent and peaches with 88 percent water. Fruits containing 87 percent water by weight include pineapple, cranberries, orange and raspberries. Apricots hold 86 percent water, while blueberries and plums contain 85 percent water. The water content for apples and pears is 84 percent. Cherries and grapes contain an average of 81 percent water. And, a banana's composition includes 74 percent water.

High Water Content Vegetables:

On top of the vegetables list are cucumber and lettuce, consisting of 96 percent water. Zucchini, radish and celery are comprised of 95 percent water. Ninety-four percent of tomato's weight is water, and green cabbage is 93 percent water. Vegetables that contain 92 percent water include cauliflower, eggplant, red cabbage, peppers and spinach. Broccoli is 91 percent water by weight. Additional healthy hydrating foods include carrots with 87 percent water and green peas and white potatoes with 79 percent water.

(http://healthyeating.sfgate.com/list-fruits-vegetable-high-water-content-8958.html)

Sports drinks with electrolytes may be useful for people doing high intensity, vigorous exercise in very hot weather, though they tend to be high in added sugars and calories.

"It's healthier to drink water while you're exercising, and then when you're done, eat a healthy snack like orange slices, bananas or a small handful of unsalted nuts," Batson said. He cautioned against fruit juices or sugary drinks, such as soda. "They can be hard on your stomach if you're dehydrated."

It's also best to avoid drinks containing caffeine, which acts as a diuretic and causes you to lose more fluids. Batson says drinking water before you exercise or go out into the sun is an important first step.

"Drinking water before is much more important," he said. "Otherwise, you're playing catch-up and your heart is straining." (www.heart.org)

Medical researcher, biochemist, and chiropractor Dr. David Williams has developed a reputation as one of the world's leading authorities on natural healing. Dr. Williams's exclusive natural treatments and remedies, often uncovered in far-flung places such as the African Bush or Australian Outback, are usually years ahead of those offered by conventional medicine. Dr. Williams's degrees and academic affiliations include multiple bachelor's degrees, a Doctor of Chiropractic from Texas Chiropractic College, and research projects at the University of Houston and the University of Texas at San Antonio.

In his valuable article *Dehydration, A Hidden Cause of Joint Pain*, Dr. Williams advises:

> Some of the primary ingredients in products that support joint health are carbohydrate and protein complexes known as glycosaminoglycans (GAGs). Along with sulfur compounds, GAGs form a thick gel-like liquid that supplies cushioning, lubrication, shock-absorption and nutrition to the cartilage in our joints. But keep in mind, they are primarily only the matrix or framework, much like a sponge. For the sponge to be "full" and "cushiony," it needs to be filled with water.

> As we age, these matrices begin to break down and our ability to keep our joints hydrated lessens. What can you do? Obviously, you need to drink plenty of water every day.

Regardless of what you may hear, 1/2 gallon a day is not unreasonable for most people.

At first, increasing the amount of water you drink may not seem like it's doing much good. In the beginning, it may just make you go to the bathroom more often, but as the matrices begin to swell again and regain their ability to retain water, that will subside. It's like trying to water a plant when the surrounding soil has dried up. When you first add water, it takes a few times before the pectin rehydrates and begins to retain the much needed water. A similar thing happens with your joints. Additionally, many of the fluids we consume nowadays act as diuretics. These include soft drinks, tea, coffee, and alcohol. Eliminating or cutting back on these can help keep you better hydrated. Lots of drugs also exhibit a diuretic effect, particularly the "water pills" given to control blood pressure.

Talk to your doctor about switching to a different blood pressure medication. (Or, better yet, use natural, drug-free therapies to lower your blood pressure.)

A diet rich in protein and fat promotes fluid loss. (Urea, a byproduct of protein, is a well-known diuretic.) Instead, try consuming more foods that are rich in complex carbohydrates. Beans, legumes, and whole grains absorb and retain water. Pretty much any high-fiber food will help tremendously, including vegetables (particularly raw), whole fruits (the pectin content in apples makes them especially helpful), and sprouted seeds. As they move through the intestinal tract, they provide a "reservoir" from which the body can pull water as it is needed. By the time most foods reach the large intestine, about the only thing being absorbed at that point is water.

Finally, if you really want to jumpstart the joint hydration process, add bone broth to your diet. The gelatin from animal bones and joints provides the GAGs, sulfur compounds, and necessary minerals in a form that's easily digested and used by the body. (www.drdavidwilliams.com)

WATERFICTION: If we consume water with increased alkalinity, we will run faster, jump higher, and live longer.

WATERFACT: When water enters the stomach, it is confronted with digestive fluid called gastric acid, aka gastric juice or stomach acid. This powerful cocktail is composed of hydrochloric acid (HCl) .05–0.1 M (roughly 5,000–10,000 parts per million) potassium chloride (KCl) and sodium chloride (NaCl). Dr. Gabe Mirkin is a graduate of Harvard University and Baylor University College of Medicine. He is board-certified in four specialties: Sports Medicine, Allergy and Immunology, Pediatrics, and Pediatric Immunology. He reports that "changing the pH of drinking water to alkaline before drinking does little or nothing to alter the pH of the blood because of the strength of stomach acid, which readily neutralizes any changes to the pH of water swallowed." (http://www.drmirkin.com/nutrition/1603.html)

Now we are arm-chair experts on the subject of what water is and what happens as we drink it, or fail to. We can feel free to initiate conversations on the subject. Now (perhaps those same) molecules of drinking water, having passed from us back into the amazing hydrologic cycle, have to find their way back into our homes via the infamous water highway: the infrastructure. How does our drinking water get to our tap? What happens under all of those mysterious man-hole covers and beyond those drains in our streets? Intriguing.

OMG, hang on tight!

Chapter

2

WATER INFRASTRUCTURE, A TRILLION DOLLAR BABY

Drinking water, whether from our faucets or bottles, gets into us humans by way of pipes. There are over 1,000,000 miles of them at last count, enough to circle the earth 60 times, according to the Environmental Protection Agency (EPA). It is difficult for us to envision what's going on in the pipes under our streets and houses, because we can't see them. We only think of this when this network fails to do something and we have to call the plumber, or the dreaded Home Owner Association (HOA) Nazis.

The prestigious Aspen Institute defines water infrastructure as "including the traditional man-made or built infrastructure components and the natural infrastructure, such as rivers, lakes, streams, groundwater aquifers, floodplains, floodways, wetlands, and the watersheds that serve or are affected by (surface) water and wastewater systems." We will also refine our understanding of the storm sewer system and the separate, but equally distinctive, sanitary sewer system under an umbrella called "infrastructure."

We only think about the pipes when a water main breaks, when the sewers back up, or when we turn on the faucet or hose and nothing comes out. The American Water Works Association (AWWA) reports that restoring existing water systems as they reach the end of their useful lives, and keeping up with population growth, will cost at least $1 trillion over the next 25 years, if we are to maintain current levels of water service. How much money is that? A trillion dollars is simply a stack of $1000 bills 63 miles high (ihtd.org). Delaying the investment can result in degrading water service, disruptions, and escalating expenditures for emergency repairs.

By contrast, the EPA "needs estimates" are more conservative, as they do not factor in population growth. Their results in 2007 found a 20-year capital investment need of almost $334.8 billion for approximately 53,000 community water systems and 21,400 not-for-profit non-community water systems (including schools and churches). Among the major necessary investments, the nation required $199 billion for transmission and distribution systems, $67 billion for treatment systems, and $39 billion for water storage.

The American Society of Civil Engineers estimates, and industry analyst Robert J. Gordon agrees, that while the cumulative cost to households from degrading water/wastewater infrastructure will add up to $59 billion (in 2010 dollars) over the period between 2013 and 2020, the cost to business will be more than double that, at $147 billion. The number of water main breaks across the country, from Syracuse to Los Angeles, is staggering: 240,000 per year, according to one estimate.

Our understanding of water infrastructure will be improved by a short history of how it was directed into our homes and gardens in ancient times. The first water infrastructure system was the aqueduct. This study of the development of aqueducts will soothe our rampant curiosity as to how water arrives in our homes and gardens today. Defined as artificial channels for water, aqueducts were built to transport water from the upper climes down to the thirsty people below. Gravity was usually the prime mover of the process, although pump technology was known. They appear in history as ornate bridges, channels or canals, or covered clay pipes. Note: this will not be on the test!

While we usually think about aqueducts as being related to ancient Rome, they were actually in use many years before the Roman Empire. Aqueducts first appeared in recorded history in Mesopotamia and on Minoan Crete around 1900 BC. Around 1400 BC, the Mycenaeans constructed aqueducts at Tiryns and Mycenae.

Long-distance aqueducts including tunnels were constructed in the Assyrian empire about 850 BC. In approximately 750 BC, sophisticated aqueducts were constructed at Babylon.

In 312 BC, Rome's first aqueduct was constructed, the 16km long Aqua Appia. Between 272 BC and 269 BC Rome's Anio Vetus aqueducts were constructed. Although not the earliest builders of aqueducts, the Romans were the most prolific, and their knowledge of construction and design of aqueducts expanded the horizons of water infrastructure. Between 144 BC and 140 BC, Rome built a 91-kilometer-long aqueduct known as the Aqua Marcia. In 50 AD, the largest Roman aqueduct, 49 meters high, was completed at Pont du Gard.

The ability to move water over distances actually sculpted the course of history by allowing the people to live farther from the source of H_2O. The necessity of water access may have also given rise to the ongoing popularity of waterfront living.

Our infrastructure discussion must include the sewer system. I carefully chose to mention our water infrastructure before the unpleasantries of sewer systems. Let's journey where Ralph Cramden's sidekick, Ed Norton of *Honeymooners* fame, went to work: the sewer. The first evidence in the history of sanitation is by way of Scotland.

About 3200 BC in Scotland, the Orkney Islands are the location of excavations that show early drainage systems. The first lavatory-like plumbing systems were fitted into recesses in the walls of homes — with drained outlets.

In Babylonia between 4000 and 2500 BC, there were storm water drain systems in the streets, with drains that were constructed of sunbaked bricks or cut stone, and some homes were connected. The need for proper disposal of human waste was not fully understood — but there was a recognition of some of the benefits (less odor, etc.) of taking these wastes away from homes. 2016 In those years, in the Mesopotamian Empire (Iraq), in some of the larger homes in Babylon people squatted over an opening in the floor of a small interior room. The wastes fell through the opening into a perforated cesspool located under the house. Unfortunately, in some parts of the world today, there is still not sufficient understanding of the need for wastewater treatment, as we found out during the 2016 Summer Olympics in Brazil in 2016, where waste is dumped directly into the ocean without treatment.

Waste disposal systems were also found to have been built between 3000 and 2000 BC by the Indus Civilization in the City of Mohenjo-daro (Pakistan). Homes had bathrooms — on the street sides — connected to sewers in streets. Bathrooms and latrines were often located next to each other, inside each home, on the street side of the home. The bathroom being located next to the latrine indicates that people understood the importance of cleanliness. Water was used for flushing.

For centuries (3000 – 100 BC), the Aegean Civilization on the Isle of Crete (Minoans) developed substantial knowledge of "hydraulics." Drainage systems of terra-cotta pipe and open-topped channelized drainage systems built of stone conveyed storm water primarily, but also human wastes.

From 2000 to 500 BC in Egypt/Palestine, certain homes of aristocrats had copper pipes that carried hot and cold water. In Egypt, certain more well-to-do homes had "toilets" — the toilets used beds of sand to catch/contain the wastes. Servants cleaned the sand regularly.

Over two thousand years ago (300 BC to 500 AD), in Greece, there were pipes of lead and bronze. Sewers in Athens delivered storm water and human wastes to a collection basin outside of town.

Not to be left out, China, between 200 BC and early AD, also had drainage technology, although it was probably only available to the highest echelon of society. The contents of a tomb of a King of the Western Han Dynasty shows the presence of an antique latrine, complete with facilities for running water, a stone seat, and a comfortable armrest.

Between 800 BC and 300 AD in Rome, public latrines were used by many people, but for the most part, human wastes were thrown into the street.

The first sewer was constructed in Rome between 800 and 735 BC. Even though not many homes were directly plumbed into the sewers, when the wastes were thrown into the street, the street washing resulted in most of the human wastes ending up in the sewers anyway!

Now we are fellow experts on the pipes that deliver water to our houses, workplaces, and work centers of our choice. We have also endured a discussion and history of waste delivery from those same places.

In the modern era the sanitary sewer system delivers its contents to a water treatment facility. We will explore the underworld of these remarkable, Dante-inspired facilities. The United States Geological Survey (USGS) will be our guide on this part of the tour (http://water.usgs.gov/edu/wwvisit. html). Please keep your hands inside of the car.

The primary treatment process:

- **Screening**: wastewater is screened for large items like wood, rocks, and the occasional unlucky creature and these items are usually sent to a landfill.
- **Pumping**: gravity is the prime mover to expedite the flow of sewage from our homes to the treatment plant. Water treatment plants, therefore, tend to be built on low ground or if above ground level the water is pumped into aeration tanks, where gravity takes over the process.
- **Aerating**: This is the act of mixing the sewage with air in an effort to remove fowl tastes and odors from the water in it. Aeration oxygenates the water and the grit settles out for removal to landfills.
- **Sludge Removal**: The water now enters sedimentation tanks where remaining sludge (the organic portion of sewage) settles out of the wastewater and is pumped out of the tanks. Some water is removed in a process called thickening and then the sludge is processed in tanks also known as digesters.
- **Removal of scum**: Lighter materials that float to the top like grease and oils, plastic and soaps are skimmed of the top. This scum is pumped to the digesters along with the sludge. Many cities add filtration.

- **Bacteria killing**: The remaining wastewater flows into a chlorine tank to kill bacteria. Other chemicals are often added. The treated water (now called effluent) is then discharged into a local river or ocean.

We now share a clear vision of most of the fairly invisible piping under our feet. Now we have to identify and envision the plumbing of the storm drains we see around our modern metropolises. This, I promise, will aid our journey into full understanding of the menagerie of pipes in our fragile drinking-water infrastructure.

Wikipedia will help, as it often does, transport us into the magic world of this new set of piping, the storm drain systems. We will emerge enlightened, never to think of all of this as "just pipes" again, and the following terms will help us distinguish between the various types of piping in our systems:

Combined Sewer: A sewer designed and intended to serve as a sanitary sewer and a storm sewer, or as an industrial sewer and a storm sewer (storm water mixed with sewage).

Storm Sewer: A sewer designed and intended to carry only storm waters, surface runoff, street wash waters, and drainage (only stormwater).

Stormwater bypass: A combined sewer discharge pipeline intended to bypass wastewater treatment plants during peak runoff events (stormwater mixed with sewage).

Roadside ditch: A roadside channel to prevent uncontrolled runoff along roadway surfaces (Only stormwater).

The objective of this jungle of concrete, overhead aquifers, lead, PVC, cast-iron, steel, and earthen piping in these two separate systems is to keep pristine and clean water flowing *to,* and the sewage properly flowing *from,* the camp.

Something was lost in translation, and pollution of our drinking water — through infrastructure design and failures — has become the norm.

The federal government did not enter the game of protecting our drinking water until 1948, with the enactment of the Federal Water Pollution Control Act of 1948 (FWPCA) was the first major law enacted by Congress to address the problems of water pollution in the United States. The Environmental Protection Agency was formed in 1970. The Clean Water Act of 1972 and the Safe Drinking Water Act of 1974 were written to monitor specific contaminants. This required close monitoring of water quality by federal, state, and municipalities for compliance. Perhaps we can appreciate the conveniences of our modern era, and perhaps the governmental intervention, however late and inept.

THE LATE, GREAT INFRASTRUCTURE

In the U.S.A. we have antiquated infrastructure. The median age of water systems in the U.S.A. is 78 years, and the median age of the sewer systems is 85 years. Due to their age, we have 240,000 water main leaks and leaky pipes draining 1.7 trillion gallons a year. The United Nations reports that water usage is doubling compared to population growth. Some pipes in use today were installed in the 1870s. In some places, the pipes appear from the outside to be fine, but what is on the corroded insides is the issue. In fact, the history and age of much of our water piping is a mystery, only unearthed when it breaks.

The U.S. Senate is in perpetual meetings on the subject of our aging water infrastructure. The Subcommittee on Water and Power is holding oversight hearing on aging water infrastructure in the U.S.A. The American Society of Civil Engineers recently gave the United States a letter grade of D or worse nearly across the board. Dam failures also compromise public safety and drinking water availability, and the deterioration of our water treatment facilities is leading to serious water-borne illness.

Is something besides pure H_2O living in there? Is something bad living in there? How worried should we be as we cautiously open our tap?

THE MASSIVE REBUILD

As alluded to above, there are varying estimates of how much it will cost to upgrade our water systems to an acceptable level. This project will not be unlike the creation of the megalithic interstate highway system conceived during the Eisenhower administration, at a cost of billions of dollars. While there was substantial debt involved in creating that system, the country received a valuable asset in return for all that money, unlike the "bad debt" bailouts that benefited the big banks during the Great Recession. There will definitely be substantial government debt incurred in this process; although we view this as good debt, as we might get a water system that lasts us another hundred years.

Sadly, as we write this, government debt in America approaches $20 trillion and counting. Will this project break the bank? Or is the bank already broken? Thankfully, some of this debt will fall upon the states and municipalities, who will need to sell tax-free municipal bonds to finance the construction of these projects. Another kick of the can down the road, as it were.

Will it cost $343 billion or $2.75 trillion, or 2017 estimates of 3.5 trillion, as some estimates indicate? Who knows? The obvious answer is that no one knows, but rest assured it will be a huge amount and will take decades of work. Who will benefit from all of this work and all of this debt? Of course, the first obvious answer is major banks, the companies that will provide the engineering, the architectural design and the manpower to get this accomplished, and perhaps the public at large via jobs.

When we look at the massive needs of these projects, there are a number of names that keep recurring in the conversation. While we are not investment advisors, we do want you to recognize the names of some of these companies, as you will undoubtedly be hearing about them in the coming years, since they will lead the way to helping us fix the problems that have been festering for many, many years.

One company that seems to be on everyone's radar is American Water Works Company, Inc., since it is the largest publicly traded water and waste water service provider in the United States. This company has been in acquisition mode for a number of years, buying up water systems. It is included in the Dow Jones Utility Average, the only water-related company in that group. The company also offers pipeline repair and upkeep, and is in the desalination and aquifer storage businesses. This company is a major global player in the water industry and has allocated billions of dollars toward infrastructure improvements and upkeep.

A similarly named, yet very different, company, American States Water Company is also a major participant in the water industry. Although it is a much smaller company than American Water Works Company, Inc., it will play a major role in the revitalization of water systems, primarily in California. This company purchases, pumps, distributes, and sells water to hundreds of thousands of people in California.

Another company frequently mentioned in the infrastructure rebuilding scenario is AECOM Technology Corp., a New York Stock Exchange listed company that offers architecture and engineering design services. Part of this multi-billion-dollar company is focused on waste water facilities, as well as related construction such as bridges and highways.

Tetra Tech Inc., a California based company, is also traded on Nasdaq, and is focused on consulting, engineering, construction, technical services, and project management in water infrastructure and resource management. With thousands of employees and billions in revenue, it's a big player in the water industry and should be another instrumental company in the revitalization of the water infrastructure over the coming years.

In the water purification segment, a name frequently mentioned is Calgon Carbon Corp. ("CCC"), another New York Stock Exchange listed company. CCC has a UV purification process, among other methods, that is highly regarded. Many new clean water regulations that took effect in 2016 will insure that CCC has some good years ahead.

Xylem is often included in discussions of rebuilding infrastructure as they are in the pump, valve, and analytic equipment business with products that move, test, and treat water. This company operates in 150 different countries, but is a New York based business, and is well positioned to take part in the biggest water infrastructure project in history.

WATERFICTION: The sanitary sewer system and the storm sewer system are the same thing. When we dispose of something down a drain it is going to get treated before being sent back into the cycle.

WATERFACT: No, they are not the same. The two systems are totally separate from each other. Our sanitary sewer system collects waste from our sinks, toilets, showers, washing machines, and dishwashers. The sanitary sewer system will then carry what was discharged to a treatment facility, where it is filtered, treated, and discharged. Our storm sewer system is designed to carry rainfall runoff and other drainage. Storm drains are part of the storm sewer system and what we see along streets and parking lots. It is not designed to carry sewage or accept hazardous wastes. The runoff is carried in underground pipes or open ditches, and discharges untreated into local streams, rivers, and other surface water bodies. Storm drain inlets are typically found built into curbs and low-lying outdoor areas. Basement floor drains are a fixture in many older buildings, and connect directly to the storm sewer system.

Now we have taken the wild ride with water molecules through the expansive infrastructure. We have cleared our understanding as to what and what not to put down what drain. Let's keep it real and talk about our obvious choice in drinking water: bottled.

Chapter

3

WATER RIDE—FROM TAPS TO BOTTLES

We buy bottled water for reasons of convenience and the perceptions of health. Drinking water from bottles follows in the footsteps of drinking from gourds and sheepskins. Drinking water is an integral part of our daily lives, and contributes, in a subtle way, to our daily craziness.

We have many choices in bottles.

Recently I purchased a Costco hot dog, and, while seated in the fine dining area there, noticed that I could buy "Kirkland Premium Water" for 25 cents, or Aquafina at $1.00 from an adjacent machine, or Dasani for $1.50 from yet another machine. My keen eye for bargains observed that, for *free*, I could essentially dispense water all day, from the soda fountain! I ultimately dealt with my temporary overwhelm by opting to drink a Pepsi with that fine hot dog.

Consumption of carbonated soft drinks has fallen to its lowest level since 1986, while global sales of bottled water products are expected to grow at a compounded annual growth rate of 8.4% from now until 2022. (http://www.briskinsights.com)

Sales of full-calorie soda in the U.S. have plummeted by more than 25% over the past 20 years. Our tastes have evolved, from sugary bottled drinks and even diet drinks, into a penchant for good, trusted water in bottles. In 2016 it is reported that bottled water sales have stolen the lead from other bottled beverages in sales.

U.S. bottled water sales leapt 6.4% in 2015, to reach $15 billion; they're projected to grow by another 34.7% by 2020. That growth includes a whopping projected sales increase of 75.1% in the segment of sparkling, mineral, and seltzer water! (www.seekingalpha.com)

There is a hearty congratulation due to someone in corporate for those achievements, I presume.

The Natural Resources Defense Council (NRDC) reports that water is:

> ... regulated by different agencies, with different missions. The U.S. Environmental Protection Agency oversees the quality of water that comes out of your tap, while the U.S. Food and Drug Administration is responsible for ensuring the safety and truthful labeling of bottled water sold nationally. States are responsible for regulating water that is both packaged and sold within its borders (which is most of the bottled-water market), but one in five states don't even bother.
>
> It's important to note that the federal government does not require bottled water to be safer than tap. In fact, just the opposite is true in many cases. Tap water in most big cities must be disinfected, filtered to remove pathogens, and tested for cryptosporidium and giardia viruses. Bottled water does not have to be tested or treated in this way. Both kinds of water are tested regularly for bacteria and most synthetic organic chemicals, but city tap is typically assessed much more frequently. For example, bottled-water plants must test for coliform bacteria just once a week; city tap needs to be tested 100 or more times a month. Limits on chemical pollution for both categories are almost

identical. The one place where bottled water might have the edge is in the case of lead; because many older homes have lead pipes, the EPA standard for tap water is less strict—one-third of the FDA's standard for lead in bottled water. (https://www.nrdc.org/stories/truth-about-tap)

The redundancy by water regulators continues unabated.

OK—but which type of water is actually safer, bottled or tap?

In 1999, after a four-year review of the bottled water industry and its safety standards, the NRDC concluded that there is no assurance that bottled water is cleaner or safer than tap. In fact, an estimated 25 percent of bottled water is really just tap water in a bottle—sometimes further treated, sometimes not.

It's rare that U. S. Food and Drug Administration (FDA) inspectors visit bottled water plants. The agency's website acknowledges that "bottled water plants generally are assigned low priority for inspection."

This lack of oversight has come at a price. Two brands have been recalled by FDA: in 2001, because of contamination with particulate matter; in 2005, due to mold and bacterial contamination.

More recently, in 2015, an E. coli scare prompted a California-based bottled water producer to recall several brands. Increasing the number of and frequency of FDA's inspections would provide a much higher chance for these types of problems to be uncovered. Some oversight of regulators and regulations could help, but that would lead to more confusion. For more information, see:

SNAFU: Situation Normal, All F....d Up.

TAFUN: Things Are Really F.....d Up Now.

FUBAR: F.....d Up Beyond All Recognition.

There are few rules in the bottled water content identity game. Bottled water companies tend to be smaller community businesses; there are a few monster players, namely Nestlé, Coke, and Pepsi.

Types of bottled water are distinct, and not just any water that happens to reside in a bottle can be sold as "bottled water." The FDA, under whose auspices this oft-maligned beverage is actually regulated as a consumer food product, mandates that the type must be stated clearly on the label.

The simple explanation, from the International Bottled Water Association, is that water can be divided into:

- Bottled Water
- Tap Water aka Municipal Water
- Filtered Water: Home or Restaurant

The source is not required to be disclosed; however, here are the "types" from http://www.bottledwater.org:

"Spring Water: derived from an underground formation from which water flows naturally to the surface of the earth. Spring water must be collected only at the spring or through a borehole tapping the underground formation feeding the spring. Spring water collected with the use of an external force must be from the same underground stratum as the spring, must have all the physical properties before treatment, and must be of the same composition and quality as the water that flows naturally to the surface of the earth.

"Purified Water: produced by distillation, deionization, reverse osmosis, or other suitable processes while meeting the definition of purified water in the United States Pharmacopoeia. Other suitable product names for bottled water treated by one of the above processes include 'distilled water' if it is produced by distillation, 'deionized water' if it is produced by deionization, or 'reverse osmosis water' if the process used is reverse osmosis. Alternatively, 'drinking water' can be used with one of the purifying terms defined above (e.g., 'purified drinking water' or 'distilled drinking water')."

To review, the FDA Standards clearly define types of water for labeling purposes:

To be called "ground water," the water must not be under the direct influence of surface water.

Water containing more than 250 parts per million of total dissolved solids is "mineral water."

"Artesian water" comes from a well tapping a confined aquifer, in which the water level stands at some height above the top of the aquifer; it may be collected with the assistance of external force to enhance the natural underground pressure.

Water that has been produced by distillation, deionization, reverse osmosis, or similar processes is "purified" or "demineralized water."

"Sparkling water" contains the same amount of carbon dioxide that it when it emerged from the source, although it may be removed and replenished in treatment.

"Spring water" must be derived from an underground formation from which water flows naturally to the Earth's surface.

"Sterile water" meets the requirements under "sterility tests" in the United States Pharmacopoeia.

"Well water" is water that has been removed from a hole bored or drilled in the ground which taps into an aquifer.

Standards of quality regulate acceptable levels of the water's turbidity, color, and odor, according to sample analysis. Exemptions are made according to aesthetically-based allowable levels, and do not relate to health concerns. An example is mineral water, which is exempt from allowable color levels.

(FDA. "21 CFR 165.110 - Requirements for Specific Standardized Beverages: Bottled Water." *Code of Federal Regulations.*)

In regards to bottled water from municipal sources, a.k.a. tap water, it is important to note that purified bottled water is not "just tap water in a bottle." Once the municipal source water enters the bottled water plant, several processes are employed to ensure that it meets the purified or sterile standard of the U.S. Pharmacopeia 23rd Revision. Those treatments can include ozonation, reverse osmosis, distillation, or de-ionization. The finished water product is then placed in a bottle under sanitary conditions and sold to the consumer.

Some critics of bottled water imply that people may be unaware they are consuming bottled water that is from a municipal water source and has been placed in a bottle without being purified. As stated above, this is not the case. If a bottled water product's source is a public water system and the finished product does not meet the FDA Standard of Identity for purified or sterile water, the product label must disclose the public water system source.

Mineral water is natural water containing not less than 250 parts per million total dissolved solids. Mineral water is distinguished from other types of bottled water by its constant level and relative proportions of mineral and trace elements at the point of emergence from the source. No minerals can be added to this product.

Sparkling bottled water is water that, after treatment and possible replacement with carbon dioxide, contains the same amount of carbon dioxide that it had as it emerged from the source. Sparkling bottled waters may be labeled as "sparkling drinking water," "sparkling mineral water," "sparkling spring water," or a similar name.

Artesian water (or Artesian well water) is water from a well that taps a confined aquifer (a water-bearing underground layer of rock or sand) in which the water level stands at some height above the top of the aquifer.

Well water is water from a hole bored, drilled, or otherwise constructed in the ground, which taps the water aquifer. (See more at http://www. bottledwater.org/types/bottled-water)

Bottled water is comprehensively regulated by the FDA. By federal law, FDA regulations governing the safety and quality of bottled water must be at least as stringent as EPA standards for tap water.

"Houston, we've had a problem here."

- first used by the crew of the Apollo 13 moon flight

Both bottled water and carbonated soda consumption averaged 38.9 gallons per capita in 2015. Bottled water consumption was 36.4 gallons per person in the U.S. Bottled water prices average an arguable $65 per gallon: more than beer, milk, or soda. This is comparable to a Starbucks triple latte with a double shot. For reference, we drank 27.6 gallons of beer and 20 gallons of milk in 2015.

"Many of the early developments in the field of chemistry can be attributed to the study of natural mineral waters and attempts to replicate them for commercial sale. Joseph Priestley, who would discover oxygen in 1775, made his first contributions to the field of chemistry by dissolving carbon dioxide in water, for which he was awarded the Copley Medal in 1773. He would go on to work with Jacob Schweppes, founder of Schweppes, in developing "aerated" waters for commercial sale." (Back, William; Landa, Edward; Meeks, Lisa. 1995. "Bottled Water, Spas, and Early Years of Water Chemistry," *Groundwater* Volume 33, Issue 4, p. 607.)

Bottled water is a part of our modern lives, and it is here to stay. What is the controversy over the ever-present bottle of water? In fact, the idea is hardly new. The ancients carries skins filled with water. Efbw.eu reports that "the bottling and commercialization of natural mineral waters first began in Europe in the mid-16th century, with mineral water from Spa in Belgium, from Vichy in France, from Ferrarelle in Italy and Apollinaris in Germany. It is said that the first mechanical corking machine was invented in France in 1840 and bottling plants emerged throughout the continent by the late 19th century. As such, other European countries also adopted the trend of bottling waters from the source, including Malvern, England's first bottled water in 1851, Germany's Appolinaris in 1892 and the Italian mineral water, San Pellegrino in 1899. Bottled waters were sold as medicinal treatment in pharmacies until the 20th century."

We are seldom without our bottles of water within reach. Bottled water is drinking water in glass or plastic, can be carbonated or not, with sizes ranging from a single serving to large containers for water coolers.

Still water distribution is led not by a single brand, but by private labels; Coca Cola follows, then Glaceau, in the U.S.A.

Top selling carbonated waters are Sparkling Ice, more private label properties, Perrier, La Croix, San Pellegrino, Glaceau Fruitwater, Topo Chico, Schweppes, Poland Springs, and Arrowhead.

So where does our brand loyalty lie, now that water sales top soda sales? *Money Magazine* reports:

> You'd think this would make the world's largest bottled water sellers happy. Instead, it's cause for great concern. Why? Joseph Agnese, an S&P Global Market Intelligence analyst, told USA Today that consumers aren't very loyal to any particular brand of water. 'In other words, water is water, and doesn't spark the same kind of heated debate that often comes up between lovers of Pepsi vs. Coke,' the article explained.
>
> The world's best-selling bottled water isn't Dasani (owned by Coca-Cola), Aquafina (PepsiCo), Poland Spring (Nestlé), or any other major brand you can think of. Instead, it's the vague category dubbed 'private label,' the all-encompassing term for generic 'store' brands.
>
> This makes sense, of course: Water is water. It's supposed to be bland, basic, and essentially flavorless. Generally speaking, you don't want it to taste different or special. So why pay extra for some 'special' brand? (Whether or not

you should pay for bottled water at all, given tap H_2O is nearly free and there are serious environmental questions raised concerning the practice of bottling, transporting, and selling water, is an entirely different discussion.)

Outside of the worries that consumers will increasingly turn to generic brands, big beverage manufacturers are concerned that the profit margins on bottled water are lower than soda. What's more, while bottled water sales are indeed rising—reportedly up 7% in 2014—the category will topple soda more quickly than expected because soda sales have been fizzling out.

Bottled water manufacturers are upset that 1) consumers aren't particularly loyal to any brands and are likely to buy whatever water is available and cheap; and 2) when consumers are buying more water, they're buying less soda. And because soda is more profitable, the Coca-Colas and Pepsis of the world would really rather be selling you soda.(http://time.com/money/4361578/bottled-water-sales-soda-brands/)

Private labels, as the largest category by sales of bottled water in the U.S., are mainly regional and privately owned. Dasani, Aquafina, and Nestlé follow in U.S. sales.

PRIVATE LABEL

The largest private label bottled water company in the U.S.A. is Niagara Bottling. "Although innovation is the key to our success at Niagara, our family tradition of high quality, value priced bottled water will never change. Niagara continues to grow and is the leading private label bottled water company in the United States…" (niagarawater.com)

DASANI® by Coke (KO)

Is described as "Purified water enhanced with minerals for a pure, fresh taste. Purified Water, Magnesium Sulfate, Potassium Chloride, Salt. ADDS

A NEGLIGIBLE AMOUNT OF SODIUM MINERALS ADDED FOR TASTE. PURIFIED BY REVERSE OSMOSIS. This product does not include ingredients sourced from genetically engineered (GE) crops, commonly known as GMOs, which the FDA regards as safe." (http://www.coca-colaproductfacts.com/en/coca-cola-products/dasani/)

AQUAFINA® by PepsiCo (PEP)

Aquafina Pure Water, the primary unflavored product produced under the Aquafina brand, is derived from local municipal tap water sources and goes through a purification process that incorporates reverse osmosis, ultraviolet and ozone sterilization. Beginning on July 27, 2007, a disclaimer was added to each bottle of Aquafina, stating the water comes from a 'public source'. Aquafina uses the term 'Purified Drinking Water' in reference to the product on its labeling in the United States. In Canada, the current 1.5 liters (51 US fl oz) bottle of water displays 'Demineralized Treated Water'. In response to concerns amongst environmental advocates who raised question over the disclosure of water sources, a PepsiCo spokeswoman stated, 'if this helps clarify the fact that the water originates from public sources, then it's a reasonable thing to do.'" (https://en.wikipedia.org/wiki/Aquafina)

S.A. (NSRGY)

The largest seller of bottled waters in the world is Nestlé, according to the Wall Street Journal, with over 60 brands. Waters North America is an affiliate of Paris-based Waters, the world's largest bottled water company.

"Regional brands in the US include Arrowhead, Calistoga, Deer Park, Ice Mountain, Ozarka, Poland Spring, and Zephyrhills. Pure Life is produced by Waters North America since 2002. Prior to that, it was known as Aberfoyle Springs and had been produced by the Aberfoyle Springs company since 1993... Their first brand was Poland Springs® brand of natural spring water, first bottled in Maine in 1845..." (https://en.wikipedia.org/wiki/Nestlé_Waters_North_America#Regional_brands)

Waters serves customers in 130 countries, with 52 well-known bottled water brands. It is, in turn, a subsidiary of the world's largest food company,

S.A, based in Vevey, Switzerland. Nestlé of North America states that they are "Promoters of Healthy Hydration."

SA is a nutrition, health, and wellness company, which manufactures, supplies, and produces prepared dishes and cooking aids, milk-based products, pharmaceuticals and ophthalmic goods, baby foods and cereals. It operates through six segments: Zone Europe; Zone Americas; Zone Asia, Oceania and Africa; Waters; Nutrition; and Other. The company was founded by Henri in 1866 and is headquartered in Vevey, Switzerland. With gross revenues in 2015 of $100.08 Billion and profits of $15.9 Billion, they employ 339,000 people."

From Nestlé: "Legend has it, the history of PERRIER goes all the way back to Hannibal crossing the Alps. It's believed that his troops prized the mineral spring's water for its clean refreshment, crisp taste and replenishing flavor. Many years later, we found those same qualities were worth sharing with North America — so we founded our company in 1976 to do just that. We started marketing PERRIER® Sparkling Natural Mineral Water in North America, and its popularity skyrocketed. Rooted in the portability of bottled water, a culture of healthy lifestyles and exercise began." (http://www.Nestle-watersna.com)

MODERN CONTROVERSY: IS WATER A RIGHT OR A PRIVILEGE?

The controversy is over whether consuming water is a right or a privilege, opening the door for charging any price the market will bear. Nestlé CEO comments:

Q. Does Chairman Peter Brabeck-Letmathe believe that water is a human right?

A. Yes. Peter Brabeck-Letmathe thinks that water is a human right and that everyone, everywhere in the world, has the right to clean, safe water for drinking and sanitation.

But what does he mean when he says that water isn't "free"?

Mr. Brabeck supports the United Nations' view that "there is enough freshwater on the planet for seven billion people, but it is distributed unevenly and too much of it is wasted, polluted and unsustainably managed."

According to UN Water, water scarcity already affects every continent. Around 1.2 billion people, or almost one-fifth of the world's population, live in areas of physical water scarcity, and 500 million people are getting closer to scarcity every day.

Mr. Brabeck has always argued that everyone should have free access to the water they need for drinking and sanitation, wherever they are in the world.

However, he does not believe it is fair that more than two billion people worldwide lack even a simple toilet, and more than one billion have no access to any kind of improved drinking source of water, while in other parts of the world people can use excess amounts of this precious and increasingly scarce resource for non-essential purposes, without bearing a cost for its infrastructure.

(http://www.nestle.com/ask-Nestle/human-rights/answers/Nestle-chairman-peter-brabeck-letmathe-believes-water-is-a-human-right)

WATERFICTION: Bottled water is better for our health and little of it is tap water.

WATERFACT: "In 1999, after a four-year review of the bottled-water industry and its safety standards, NRDC concluded that there is no assurance that bottled water is cleaner or safer than tap. In fact, an estimated 25 percent or more of bottled water is really just tap water in a bottle—sometimes further treated, sometimes not.

"Of the 1,000 bottles tested, the majority proved to be relatively clean and pure. About 22 percent of the brands tested contained chemicals at levels above state health limits in at least one sample. If consumed over a long period of time, some of those contaminants could cause

cancer or other health problems for people with weakened immune systems..." (www.nrdc.org)

Both Aquafina, from PepsiCo, and Dasani, from The Coca-Cola Company, originate from municipal water systems. However, according to the FDA, about 75 percent of bottled water sold in the U.S. comes from other sources, including "natural underground sources, which include rivers, lakes, springs and artesian wells." (Lempert, Phil. Is your bottled water coming from a faucet? MSNBC.com, July 21, 2004.)

We have learned about getting our water from taps and bottles, and that perhaps the bottles contain tap water. We know who many of the top players are in the bottled water game and all about the controversy over our right or privilege to drink it.

Now we are going to find out what terrible things can happen to water along the path to grandma's house.

Chapter

4

WATER TOXICITY, GOOD WATER GONE ROGUE

We count on the purity and sanctity of our tap and bottled water, and we rely on the government to, somehow, monitor and police our drinking water supply. How is it that our water has become toxic? Our drinking water originates from ground water and surface sources. The government, in the guise of the Environmental Protection Agency (EPA), sets acceptable limits on the presence of over 90 chemicals of concern. Understanding what the EPA is doing naturally involves bracing ourselves for the onslaught of acronyms that always follow our trusted government's method of communicating reassurances about matters of public safety:

> EPA has established National Primary Drinking Water Regulations (NPDWRs). National Primary Drinking Water Regulations are legally enforceable standards that apply to public water systems. These standards protect drinking water quality by limiting the levels of specific contaminants that can adversely affect public health and which are known or anticipated to occur in public water supplies. (NPDWRs) that set mandatory water quality standards for drinking water contaminants. These are

enforceable standards called 'maximum contaminant level (MCL).'

The highest level of a contaminant that is allowed in drinking water as delineated by the National Primary Drinking Water Regulations. These levels are based on consideration of health risks, technical feasibility of treatment, and cost-benefit analysis.

'Maximum Contaminate Levels' (MCLs) which are established to protect the public against consumption of drinking water contaminants that present a risk to human health. An MCL is the maximum allowable amount of a contaminant in drinking water which is delivered to the consumer.

In addition, EPA has established National Secondary Drinking Water Regulations (NSDWRs) that set non-mandatory water quality standards for 15 contaminants. EPA does not enforce these 'secondary maximum contaminant levels' (SMCLs). They are established only as guidelines to assist public water systems in managing their drinking water for aesthetic considerations, such as taste, color, and odor. These contaminants are not considered to present a risk to human health at the SMCL. (http://www. epa.gov)

In addition to the EPA monitored chemicals, us humans, our pets, and agriculture also introduce toxins into our drinking water.

Before we ascend further into the abyss of exactly which chemicals are being identified and regulated by big government, here is a short list of serious drinking water offenders. We will continue to refine our understanding of the scope of our drinking water toxicity in the U.S.A. by focusing on top water concerns, then continue our ascent into the murk.

PFASs, PHARMACEUTICALS, ASBESTOS, ARSENIC, RADIO-ACTIVITY, FLUORIDE, CHROMIUM

PFASs

Levels of a widely used class of industrial chemicals linked with cancer and other health problems — polyfluoroalkyl and perfluoroalkyl substances (PFASs) — exceed federally recommended safety levels in public drinking water supplies for six million people in the U.S., according to a 2016 study led by researchers from Harvard T.H. Chan School of Public Health and the Harvard John A. Paulson School of Engineering and Applied Sciences (SEAS).

"For many years, chemicals with unknown toxicities, such as PFASs, were allowed to be used and released to the environment, and we now have to face the severe consequences," said lead author Xindi Hu, a doctoral student in the Department of Environmental Health at Harvard Chan School and Environmental Science and Engineering at SEAS. "In addition, the actual number of people exposed may be even higher than our study found, because government data for levels of these compounds in drinking water is lacking for almost a third of the U.S. population — about 100 million people."

PFASs have been used over the past 60 years in industrial and commercial products ranging from food wrappers, to clothing, to pots and pans. They have been linked with cancer, hormone disruption, high cholesterol, and obesity. Although several major manufacturers have discontinued the use of some PFASs, the chemicals continue to persist in people and wildlife. Drinking water is one of the main routes through which people can be exposed.

The researchers looked at concentrations of six types of PFASs in drinking water supplies, using data from more than 36,000 water samples collected nationwide by the EPA from 2013-2015. They also looked at industrial sites that manufacture or use PFASs; at military fire training sites and civilian airports where fire-fighting foam containing PFASs is used; and at wastewater treatment plants. Discharges from these plants — which are unable to remove PFASs from wastewater by standard treatment methods

— could contaminate groundwater. So could the sludge that the plants generate, which is frequently used as fertilizer.

The study found that PFASs were detectable at the minimum reporting levels required by the EPA in 194 out of 4,864 water supplies in 33 states across the U.S. Drinking water from 13 states accounted for 75% of the detections, including, in order of frequency of detection, California, New Jersey, North Carolina, Alabama, Florida, Pennsylvania, Ohio, New York, Georgia, Minnesota, Arizona, Massachusetts, and Illinois.

Sixty-six of the public water supplies examined, serving six million people, had at least one water sample that measured at or above the EPA safety limit of 70 parts per trillion (ng/L) for two types of PFASs, perfluorooctanesulfonic acid (PFOS), and perfluorooctanoic acid (PFOA). Concentrations ranged as high as 349 ng/L for PFOA (Warminster, PA) and 1,800 ng/L for PFOS (Newark, DE).

The highest levels of PFASs were detected in watersheds near industrial sites, military bases, and wastewater treatment plants — all places where these chemicals may be used or found.

"These compounds are potent immunotoxins in children and recent work suggests drinking water safety levels should be much lower than the provisional guidelines established by EPA," said Elsie Sunderland, senior author of the study and associate professor in both the Harvard Chan School and SEAS." (https://www.sciencedaily.com/releases/2016/08/160809121418.htm)

PHARMACEUTICALS IN OUR WATER

The number of retail drug prescriptions filled in 2015 in the U.S.A., to humans, was 4,065,175,000. Recent studies have discovered pharmaceuticals in our drinking water as a result of some portion of all of them having been flushed by or excreted by us humans. Note that excretion is a process whereby drugs pass from our bodies to the external environment. (A 2007 study in California found that over 50% of all drugs were tossed back into the environment, unused.) Drugs vary greatly as to how long they remain in us, because of their different bonds to our tissue components. Our metabolic rate and tissue redistribution will also greatly affect the efficacy of a drug, and — more to our interest here — the rate of elimination into the environment.

"The two trillion pounds of animal waste generated by large-scale poultry and livestock operations in this country is laced with hormones and antibiotics fed to animals to make them grow faster and to keep them from getting sick. Inevitably, some of those hormones and antibiotics leach into groundwater or get into waterways." (http://www.health.harvard.edu/ newsletter_article/drugs-in-the-water)

Hospitals and pharmaceutical factories are also huge contributors to the toxification of our drinking water. The fact that many pharmaceutical and recreational drugs are synthetic introduces a bewildering complexity of hybrid substances into our drinking water world. These chemicals are like needles in haystacks to identify and monitor, despite advances in chemical spectral analytics. If a researcher is not specifically looking for a particular chemical, it will not be identified in the report. This is much like a pre-employment drug test, in which they (and you) must know in advance exactly what they are looking for.

There is a school of thought that the identification and regulation of new drugs and toxic chemicals in our beleaguered drinking water supply in the U.S.A. is scrupulously avoided by regulators because of the political nightmares lurking under that waterbed. It is rumored that there is, unavoidably, some trace of recreational drugs therein. Frightening indeed.

How big is the problem? The Harvard report, cited above states that:

> A study conducted by the U.S. Geological Survey in 1999 and 2000 found measurable amounts of one or more medications in 80% of the water samples drawn from a network of 139 streams in 30 states. The drugs identified included a witches' brew of antibiotics, antidepressants, blood thinners, heart medications (ACE inhibitors, calcium-channel blockers, digoxin), hormones (estrogen, progesterone, testosterone), and painkillers. Scores of studies have been done since. Other legal drugs that have been found include caffeine (which, of course, comes from

many other sources besides medications); carbamazepine, an anti seizure drug; fibrates, which improve cholesterol levels; and some fragrance chemicals (galaxolide and tonalide)...

ASBESTOS

Asbestos related diseases characteristically develop over a long period of time. The first symptoms may not appear for anything from 10 to 50 years. Peak mortality rates are expected between the years 2010 and 2020.

The list of asbestos-related diseases includes:

1. Mesothelioma
2. Asbestosis
3. Lung Cancer
4. Laryngeal Cancer
5. Ovarian Cancer
6. Testes Cancer
7. Pleural plaques
8. Pleural thickening
9. Pleural effusion

Asbestos first showed up in cement pipes carrying drinking water in 1931, having been in production since 1906. The pipes were made from a mixture of Portland Cement and asbestos fiber, used to make the pipe resistant to corrosion. The American Water Works Association set standards by 1953 governing the use of asbestos pipes in municipal water systems in the U.S.A. With a projected life of 70 years, many of these pipes remain in use today. As the pipes deteriorate they leach measurable asbestos into the water: "There is as much as 400,000 miles of asbestos pipe in use in the USA." (http://www.haz-mat.ca/asbestos-removal/asbestos/ et al)

A report from Detroit showed more than 3 million asbestos fibers in a single quart of tap water. It is unclear what health risks a single cup of water containing fibers will cause.

Asbestos is known to be a human carcinogen. Asbestos is a group of minerals that occur naturally as bundles of fibers. These fibers are found in soil and rocks in many parts of the world. They are made mainly of silicon and oxygen, but they also contain other elements. Asbestos does not dissolve in water. There are 2 main types of asbestos:

- Chrysotile asbestos, also known as white asbestos, is the most common type of asbestos in industrial applications. When looked at under the microscope, chrysotile asbestos fibers wrap around themselves in a spiral, which is why this form of asbestos is also called serpentine or curly asbestos. An area that included Everett, Washington, was selected for a recent study because of the unusually high concentration of chrysotile asbestos in drinking water from the Sultan River. (ncbi.nih.gov)
- Amphibole asbestos fibers are straight and needle-like. There are several types of amphibole fibers, including amosite (brown asbestos), crocidolite (blue asbestos), tremolite, actinolite, and anthophyllite. "Iron ore called taconite is mined in the Biwabik Iron Formation in the Eastern Mesabi region of the Mesabi Range, in eastern Minnesota. After mining, ore is shipped to Silver Bay, Minnesota for processing and wet magnetic extraction. Tailings from the process are dumped, as a slurry, into a man-made containment delta constructed in Lake Superior. Submicroscopic amphibole fibers and/or cleavage fragments, a component of the gangue, apparently escape from the delta at Silver Bay, and enter Lake Superior. (http://www.ncbi.nlm.nih.gov/pubmed/294208)

The main risk from asbestos cement pipes comes from the possibility of ingesting water contaminated with loose fibers. Individuals who lived in areas where transite pipe was used in the water system may be at enhanced risk of developing peritoneal mesothelioma from the ingestion of asbestos material.

Read more on asbestos: http://www.mesothelioma.com/asbestos-exposure/products/cement-pipe/

ARSENIC

The following signs and symptoms are associated in more severe cases of arsenic poisoning:

- metallic taste in the mouth
- mouth produces excess saliva
- problems swallowing
- blood in the urine
- cramping muscles
- loss of hair
- stomach cramps
- convulsions
- excessive sweating
- breath smells like garlic
- vomiting
- diarrhea

Arsenic poisoning typically affects the skin, liver, lungs and kidneys — hence, the severity of the symptoms. The final stage of the poisoning causes the patient to suffer seizures and go into shock, this could lead to death or coma (and likely subsequent death). (http://www.medicalnewstoday.com/articles/241860.php)

In 2000, nearly 36 million Americans drank water containing arsenic at or above 3 parts per billion — the level NRDC had urged be established as a drinking water standard. The EPA had delayed and delayed updating the arsenic standard that was originally issued in the 1960s, but updated the arsenic number based on modern science in the early 2000s.

> Water utilities measure arsenic at the entry point to a distribution system for compliance determinations. When arsenic level in the treated water supply is below the 10 parts per billion drinking water standard, that particular drinking water source is generally considered safe for human consumption at the tap. Just what is arsenic and how did it get near our drinking waters?

Arsenic is released to the environment from a variety of natural and anthropogenic sources. In the environment, arsenic occurs in rocks, soil, water, air, and in biota. Average concentrations in the earth's crust reportedly range from 1.5 to 5 mg/kg *(Cullen and Reimer, 1989)*. Higher concentrations are found in some igneous and sedimentary rocks, particularly in iron and manganese ores (Welch et al., 1988). In addition, a variety of common minerals contain arsenic, of which the most important are arsenopyrite (FeAsS), realgar (AsS), and orpiment (As2S3). Natural concentrations of arsenic in soil typically range from 0.1 to 40 mg/kg, with an average concentration of 5 to 6 mg/kg (National Academy of Sciences (NAS), 1977). Through erosion, dissolution, and weathering, arsenic can be released to ground water or surface water. Geothermal waters can be sources of arsenic in ground water, particularly in the Western United States (Nimick et al., 1998, Welch et al., 1988).

Other natural sources include volcanism and forest fires. Anthropogenic sources of arsenic relate to its use in the lumber, agriculture, livestock, and general industries. Most agricultural uses of arsenic are banned in the United States. However, organic arsenic is a constituent of the organic herbicides monosodium methanearsonate (MSMA) and disodium methanearsonate (DSMA), which are currently applied to cotton fields as herbicides (Jordan et al., 1997). Organic arsenic is also a constituent of feed additives for poultry and swine, and appears to concentrate in the resultant animal wastes (NAS, 1977).

The potential impact of arsenic in animal wastes used to fertilize crops is uncertain. Most of the arsenic used in the United States is for the production of chromated copper arsenate (CCA), the wood preservative *(Reese, 1998)*. CCA is used to pressure treat lumber and is classified as a restricted use pesticide by the USEPA. A significant industrial use of arsenic is the production of lead-acid batteries, while small amounts of very pure arsenic metal are used to produce the semiconductor crystalline gallium arsenide, which is used in computers and other electronic applications.

Arsenic is also released from industrial processes, including the burning of fuels and wastes, mining and smelting, pulp and paper production, glass manufacturing, and cement manufacturing (USEPA, 1998b). In addition, past waste disposal sites may be contaminated with arsenic. Arsenic is a contaminant of concern at 916 of the 1,467 sites on the National Priorities List (NPL) *(Agency for Toxic Substances and Disease Registry (ATSDR), 1998)*. Sites included on the NPL have the potential to release contaminants to ground water or surface water in the vicinity of the site. Anthropogenic releases of arsenic to the environment can be estimated from Toxics Release Inventory (TRI) data. These data indicate that 7,947,012 pounds of arsenic and arsenic containing compounds were released to the environment in 1997, a significant increase from 3,536,467 pounds in 1995 *(USEPA, 1999a)*. The increase primarily occurred at one facility, where arsenic on-site land releases increased by 3.58 million pounds from 1995 to 1997 because of a change in the facility's smelting process that was implemented to reduce sulfur dioxide emissions.

The TRI data do omit some potentially significant arsenic sources, including arsenic associated with the application of herbicides and fertilizers and arsenic released from mining facilities and electric utilities. Arsenic Fate and Transport Once arsenic released from natural or anthropogenic sources enters ground water or surface water, a variety of processes affect its fate and transport. These include oxidation reduction reactions, transformations, ligand exchange, and biotransformations. The factors that affect these reactions include the oxidation state of the arsenic, oxidation-reduction potential (Eh), pH, concentrations of iron, metal sulfides, and sulfides, temperature, salinity, and the distribution and composition of biota...

Scales on pipes and other components in distribution systems may contain relatively high arsenic concentrations, in some cases consumer tap water may exceed the drinking water standard for arsenic and become a health threat to consumers. But the truth is until there is new data from the water utility community, the relative amounts of arsenic perhaps being drank by the population is not known. (http://www.freedrinkingwater.com)

RADIOACTIVITY

On March 11, 2011, a 9.0 magnitude earthquake struck just off the coast of Honshu Island, Japan, which caused the automatic shutdown of three of the six reactors located at the Fukushima power plant. Routine maintenance of the three other reactors was being performed at that time and they were offline. The tremor isolated the plant from the power grid.

A 46-foot tsunami struck the plant and breached the protective seawall. The emergency power used for reactor cooling is washed away. In April, the Japanese government officially raised Fukushima to The International Nuclear and Radiological Event (INES) Level 7, the same as Chernobyl.

The effects, handling, and reporting of this disaster and subsequent water radiation levels and environmental consequences for drinking water in the U.S. are hotly contested.

There are detectable amounts of radiation in the environment, occurring naturally in soil, rocks, water, air, and vegetation, from which it is inhaled and ingested into the body. Cosmic radiation emanates from space. Radioactive particles (radionuclides) can also spread easily through underground water systems used to capture drinking water.

Radionuclide is defined as "an unstable form of a chemical element that radioactively delays, resulting in the emission of nuclear radiation." (medicinenet.com)

Radionuclides in drinking water include isotopes of uranium, radium, radon, and others. Cesium and iodine are also of concern and they are from manmade nuclear reactions. Radioactive pollution is also cumulative: it builds up in the body over time. Drinking is a primary method of exposure to radioactivity.

Maximum uranium levels are set by the EPA. At some levels these radioactive particles are known to cause kidney damage and increase risk of certain cancers. Radioactive iodine collects in the thyroid and can cause cancer there as it decays.

FLUORIDE (addressed more fully in Chapter 7)

Public water fluoridation was first practiced in 1945 in the U.S. As of 2012, 25 countries have artificial water fluoridation to varying degrees; 11 of them have more than 50% of their population drinking fluoridated water. A further 28 countries have water that is naturally fluoridated, though in many of them the fluoride is above the recommended safe level. As of 2012 about 435 million people worldwide received water fluoridated at the recommended level (i.e., about 5.4% of the global population). About 214 million of them are living in the United States.

Total US population, persons	318,857,056
US population on community water systems (CWS), persons	286,756,186
Total US population on fluoridated drinking water systems, persons	214,213,860
Percentage of US population receiving fluoridated water	67.2%

For a complete listing of fluoridation, by state: http://www.cdc.gov/fluoridation/statistics/2014stats.htm

CHROMIUM

In 2010 the Environmental Working Group (EWG) found excessive levels of chromium 6, a carcinogen, in the water supply of 31 U.S. cities. Exposure to chromium 6 causes a long list of conditions, including stomach cancer, kidney failure, renal and liver failure, premature dementia, and allergic contact dermatitis.

Chromates are often used to make leather goods, mortar, and paints, and they leach from these industrial processes into groundwater and soil, eventually ending up in our water.

LEAD (addressed more fully in Chapter 6)

Particularly toxic to children, it interferes with the development of the nervous system and can cause anemia, seizures and even death. Lead is found in copper plumbing; almost all houses built before 1986 likely have lead-soldered copper water pipes.

The signs and symptoms of lead poisoning in children may include:

- Developmental delay
- Learning difficulties
- Irritability
- Loss of appetite
- Weight loss
- Sluggishness and fatigue
- Abdominal pain
- Vomiting
- Constipation
- Hearing loss

Babies who are exposed to lead before birth may experience:

- Learning difficulties
- Slowed growth

Although children are primarily at risk, lead poisoning is also dangerous for adults. Signs and symptoms in adults may include:

- High blood pressure
- Abdominal pain
- Constipation
- Joint pains
- Muscle pain
- Declines in mental functioning

- Pain, numbness or tingling of the extremities
- Headache
- Memory loss
- Mood disorders
- Reduced sperm count, abnormal sperm
- Miscarriage or premature birth in pregnant women (http://www.mayoclinic.org/ et al)

Scientific America reports that:

> Researchers from the U.S. Geological Survey and the Environmental Protection Agency analyzed single samples of untreated and treated water from 25 U.S. utilities who voluntarily participated in the project. Twenty-one contaminants were detected – mostly in low concentrations of parts per billion– in treated drinking water from at least nine of the utilities. Eighteen of the chemicals are not regulated under the federal Safe Drinking Water Act so utilities do not have to meet any limit or even monitor for them...

This means that, in this particular study, researchers were looking for toxins that are not normally monitored by the EPA, but are toxins nevertheless, and they are present in many municipal water systems. The effect of these toxic chemicals, in these quantities, and mixed with other contaminants, is the unknown. This is another serious consideration as we cautiously open our taps.

How else do toxic chemicals find their way into our personal water supply? The infrastructure, discussed at length in Chapter 2, carries sewage and water run-off and picks up a host of undesirables along the way. Many well-meaning municipal water plants, built long ago, are overwhelmed in their efforts to capture these substances in recycling for consumption. There is new meaning in the familiar sounding "Sewage and Water Board."

Yes, there is every likelihood that there is commingling, and the name is no coincidence. Perhaps the word water should have come first, to make the idea less graphic. Water "reuse" is a term used in explaining the delicate subject of reclamation of drinking water from sewage.

Rainfall can toxify our drinking water! The term "acid rain" is a serious indictment against even the most innocent of afternoon April showers. It refers to the pH of rain water outside, while the near-hostile debate over the acidity and alkalinity of drinking water rages on indoors. pH is a numeric indicator for the acidity of a substance and is determined by the number of free hydrogen ions (H+) present. A comparison of the number of hydrogen (H+) ions and the number of hydroxide (OH-) ions equals "pH" and when equal the water is said to be neutral. This will result in a measured pH of approximately 7. With a scale range of 0-14, a number above 7 is alkaline or basic, and below 7 is acidic.

Air pollutants of dust, smoke, and smog are stirred up by air currents and deposited on earth or surface water by rainfall. Rainfall is slightly acidic due to the carbonic acid from carbon dioxide in atmosphere. "Acid rain" is caused when sulfur dioxide (SO_2) and nitrogen oxides** emanating from industrial emissions and auto exhausts are picked up by rain as weak sulfuric and nitric acid.

Salty oceans make up 97% of the water on earth: that totals 365.8 trillion million gallons. The remaining 3% of fresh water would measure 10 trillion million gallons, in layman's terms. How could there ever be a problem finding clean sources? Maintaining sources of clean drinking water is the bane of our modern world, with the CDC reporting that "waterborne diseases are caused by pathogenic microbes that can be directly spread through contaminated water... The usual cause of death is dehydration. Most cases of diarrheal illness and death occur in developing countries because of unsafe water, poor sanitation, and insufficient hygiene... These diseases can (also) cause malnutrition, skin infections, and organ damage..." Water-borne diseases are any illness caused by drinking water contaminated by human or animal feces, which contain pathogenic microorganisms. Bad juju.

The "point of use" concept of water cleanliness comes into play. The water must start out clean at the source and remain that way, getting all the way into us humans, to be considered nontoxic or pure. In the developing world, the pipes, treatment facilities, bottles, glasses, or jugs may be contaminated. In our modern world, the inside of the pipes are the main infrastructure culprit.

In the U.S. we have antiquated infrastructure (see Chapter 2) that is incapable of protecting our drinking water. The many miles of still-in-place asbestos-laden pipes corrode and give way to leaching into our water supply. The median age of water systems in the U.S. is 78 years, and median age of the sewer system is 85 years, with 240,000 water main leaks and leaky pipes draining 1.7 trillion gallons a year. United Nations reports that water usage is doubling compared to population growth. Some of the pipes in use today have been in the ground since the Civil War era! Jupiter, Florida reports an actual wooden feeder pipe still in service.

The Water and Wastewater Equipment Manufacturers Association (WWEMA) participated in several of the 2016 Infrastructure Week events, beginning with the kick-off event held at the U.S. Chamber of Commerce, and culminating with the May 18 Advocacy Day on the Hill and a reception hosted by the U.S. Water Alliance.

WWEMA was one of 150 affiliate organizations that joined the steering committee members and Congressional co-chairs to spread the word that "Infrastructure Matters." Mayors, business leaders, manufacturers, utilities, and industry organizations across all infrastructure came together in Washington, D.C., and held events across the country to emphasize the importance of building/rebuilding our nation's infrastructure.

The U.S. Senate is in perpetual debate on the shape and rebuilding of the water infrastructure. The Subcommittee on Water and Power is holding oversight hearings on aging water infrastructure across the country. Dam failures also compromise public safety and water treatment facilities deteriorating can lead to water borne illness.

> The Water Resources Development Act of 2016 S. 2848 was recently introduced by U. S. Senators Jim Inhofe (R-Okla.), Chairman of the U.S. Senate Environment and Public Works (EPW) Committee, and Barbara Boxer

(D-CA) ranking member of the Senate EPW Committee summarized here:

The Water Resources Development Act of 2016 (WRDA) authorizes 25 critical Army Corps projects in 17 states. These projects, which have undergone Congressional scrutiny and have completed reports of the Chief of Engineers, will strengthen our nation's infrastructure to protect lives and property, restore vital ecosystems to preserve our natural heritage, and maintain navigation routes for commerce and the movement of goods to keep us competitive in the global marketplace.

The bill provides critical investment in the country's aging drinking water and wastewater infrastructure, assists poor and disadvantaged communities in meeting public health standards under the Clean Water Act and Safe Drinking Water Act, and promotes innovative technologies to address drought and other critical water resource needs. The bill also responds to the drinking water crisis in Flint, Michigan, by providing emergency assistance to Flint and other similar communities.... facing drinking water contamination.

The bill:

- Invests in the Nation's Ports and Inland Waterways to Improve Commerce
- Improves Flood Protection and Safety for Communities
- Restores Ecosystems and Promotes Public Access for Recreation
- Addresses High Priority, Regional Water Resources Issues
- Streamlines Reviews and Increases Local Participation
- Promotes Innovative Technologies to Address Water Resources Challenges
- Increases Flexibility and Federal Assistance to Address Drought

- Provides Essential Investment in Drinking Water and Wastewater Infrastructure (http://www.epw.senate.gov/public/_cache/files/797e0d1b-abf5-4df7-869a-3836356cd3c6/wrda-2016-highlights.pdf)

As Led Zeppelin sang: "When the levee breaks, mama, you got to move."

We have vague notions that the government is disingenuous in their efforts to keep our water safe and pure, more bent on regulating than correcting. These feelings are sort of like a mild migraine: we don't know exactly when it started, but there it is.

As our study continues we cannot help but recognize the sheer number of water toxins that our well-intended H_2O is contending with. We have learned that genteel molecules of water are floating upwards from the pristine oceans in the evaporative process. The formation of clouds is also aided by transpiration, as the leaves of plants make their contribution to the hydrologic cycle. We envision the gentle rain that follows as the water droplets gently fall onto the patiently waiting earth. From there all hell breaks loose! A hail-storm of drinking water toxicity goes on the full offensive!

> **"High and fine literature is wine, and mine is only water, but everyone likes water."**
>
> *- Mark Twain*

The challenge of clean water and control of the resulting waterborne diseases is twofold: access to upgraded water sources, and open toilet practices. According to *The Guardian,* nearly 100 million people go to the toilet outside, contaminating drinking water sources, and spreading diseases such as cholera, diarrhea, dysentery, hepatitis A, and typhoid. Globally 2.4 billion people lack sanitary water, defined as one that hygienically separates human waste from human contact.

These stunning statistics from the developing world makes it particularly difficult for us to accept the notion that there are any inferiorities in our modern municipal water systems. Many of the pipes were laid over 100 years ago! What evil lurks there?

The Safe Drinking Water Act (SDWA) is the federal law that protects public drinking water supplies throughout the nation. Under the SDWA, the EPA sets standards for drinking water quality and, with its partners, implements various technical and financial programs to ensure drinking water safety.

There is a vague and carefully planted idea that a filter on a faucet will eliminate toxins, and to some extent, this is a fact. The question is: what are we are filtering for and how small is it?

Just when we thought everything in water was perfectly identified and regulated, science vastly improved their ability to "look more closely." Lawrence Berkeley National Labs (who knew?) just turned on a $27 million electron microscope. With the ability to make images to a resolution of half the width of a hydrogen atom this makes it the most powerful microscope in the world.

Along the way to this present-day development, the ability to identify the smallest of offenders in the water-world have evolved steadily since Zaccharias Janssen invented the microscope in 1590. The identifying of additional rogue elements in drinking water has been a process in which the government has always appeared to be quite satisfied with the culprits they were already tracking.

Science and the water consuming public appeared to go on a rampage of discovery, and a host of new suspect chemicals are now being exposed in the bright light of spectral analysis, identified, in parts per million (ppm), billion (ppb), and trillion (ppt). How could these culprits have escaped detection? Well, it appears that one must tell the now progressively mega-powerful microscopes what to look for beforehand!

To further understand the length and breadth of the US water purity problem an exhaustive list of *Regulation Development for Drinking Water Contaminants*: has been included in the notes section, for your reference: see the *Code of Federal Regulations: Title 40 – Protection of the Environment.*

The National Primary Drinking Water Regulations (NPDWRs, or primary standards) are legally enforceable standards that apply to public water systems. Primary standards protect public health by limiting the levels of contaminants in drinking water. reference:

(https://www.epa.gov/ground-water-and-drinking-water/table-regulated-drinking-water-contaminants)

Now we have explored the realities of chemicals in our drinking water. We have identified many of the EPA-monitored pollutants that threaten our tap water, and how our aging infrastructure contributes to this dilemma. The geographic diversity, within the US, of many of the pollutants identified further frustrates our efforts to understand what, exactly, we are "solving for."

What exactly are we are chasing in the dog fight for pure drinking water? Who are our enemies? Allies? What are our purification alternatives? Some of the chemicals are more dangerous than others: we will discuss them here, and, more importantly, how we can remove them. Read on...

WATERFICTION: Our government knows the identity of the toxins in our drinking water, and protects us at our point-of-use.

WATERFACT: Our government monitors and regulates some toxins in our drinking water, but the presence of many toxins is unknown, unmonitored, and the identities of many hybrid threats are totally unidentified. Their responsibility ends at our water meter.

Chapter

5

WATER AGITATION, GETTING FRACKED

TRADING WATER FOR OIL AND GAS

What in the world does producing oil and gas from the underground have to do with our drinking water?

Fracking is short for hydrofracking and yes, the "hydro" designation involves our water. It is no coincidence that water's intimate involvement with the process is often hidden, even in the name! Defined as "a well-stimulation technique in which rock is fractured by a pressurized liquid," other names for the process are Hydrofracking, Hydraulic Fracturing, and Hydro fracturing.

> The process involves the high-pressure injection of 'fracking fluid' (primarily water, containing sand or other proppants suspended with the aid of thickening agents) into a wellbore to create cracks in the deep-rock formations through which natural gas, petroleum, and brine will flow more freely. When the hydraulic pressure is removed from the well, small grains of hydraulic fracturing proppants (either sand or aluminum oxide) hold the fractures open.

Hydraulic fracturing began as an experiment in 1947, and the first commercially successful application followed in 1950. As of 2012, 2.5 million 'frac jobs' had been performed worldwide on oil and gas wells; over one million of those within the U.S.

Such treatment is generally necessary to achieve adequate flow rates in shale gas, tight gas, tight oil, and coal seam gas wells.

Hydrofracking is of great concern because of the possibility of its negative affect on our drinking water purity and progressive drinking water scarcity. The amount of water required to hydraulically fracture oil and gas wells varies widely across the country. USGS research found that water volumes for hydraulic fracturing averaged within watersheds across the United States range from as little as 2,600 gallons to as much as 9.7 million gallons per well.

The opposite side of the argument is that the cost-benefit ratio of fracking is well worth the risk to the environment of polluting the ground water, and of removal of water for the process.

This very old process causes fractures that allow the toxic chemicals used in the process to find their way into surface and ground water. There is sensitive geology involved, and the other point of offense in fracking is the dumping of chemicals pumped down into the earth, inevitably finding its way into our drinking water … or not.

According to environmentalamerica.com:

> Drinking water contamination – fracking brings with it the potential for spills, blowouts and well failures that contaminate groundwater supplies. Cleanup of drinking water contamination is so expensive that it is rarely even attempted. In Dimock, Pennsylvania, Cabot Oil & Gas reported having spent $109,000 on systems to remove methane from well water for 14 local households, while in Colorado, cleanup of an underground gas seep has been

ongoing for eight years at a cost of hundreds of thousands of dollars, if not more.

The provision of temporary replacement water supplies is also expensive. Cabot Oil & Gas reported having spent at least $193,000 on replacement water for homes with contaminated water in Dimock, Pennsylvania. Fracking can also pollute drinking water sources for major municipal systems, increasing water treatment costs. If fracking were to degrade the New York City watershed with sediment or other pollution, construction of a filtration plant would cost approximately $6 billion...

Environmental Science and Technology published a Stanford University study stating that "it is perfectly legal to inject stimulation fluids into underground drinking water. This may be causing widespread impacts on drinking water resources."

As of 2012, 2.5 million hydraulic fracturing jobs have been performed on oil and gas wells worldwide, more than one million of them in the United States.

Uranium Energy Corporation is planning to use hydraulic fracturing to mine uranium, with additional threats to our drinking water supply. Fracking for uranium involves injecting oxygenated water (to increase solubility) to dissolve the uranium, then pumping the solution back up to the surface.

Proponents of hydraulic fracturing point to the economic benefits from the vast amounts of formerly inaccessible hydrocarbons the process can extract.

Opponents point to potential environmental effects, including contamination of ground water, depletion of fresh water, risks to air quality, noise pollution, the migration of gases and hydraulic fracturing chemicals to the surface, surface contamination from spills and flow-back, and the health effects of these.

The Pros of Fracking:

- Greatly reduces our dependence on foreign oil.
- Revives old wells making production possible.
- Increases our reserves.
- Creates jobs.

Although there is an array of benefits, many are concerned about the environmental impact natural gas fracking may have on our environment.

The cons of fracking:

- The emissions from fracking are double that of coal and could severely increase air pollution around the site.
- Fracking consumes a large amount of water, with some wells requiring between one and eight million gallons of water to crack the rock. In some cases, only 30-50% of the water is recovered.
- Proprietary chemicals are used in the fracking process, sometimes containing nearly 600 different chemicals. This can certainly be a concern for the personnel working at the site, along with the tainted recovered water.
- It has been reported that methane levels in ground water near fracking sites have been up to 17 times higher than normal. This will have a severe impact on local residents.

Over 30% of our natural gas is obtained by hydraulic fracking, with 45% of gas coming from the process by 2035, according to The Energy Information Administration.

For these reasons hydraulic fracturing has come under international scrutiny, with some countries protecting it, and others suspending or banning it.

The EPA describes the process and potential effects of the process on drinking water:

Stage 1: Water Acquisition

- Large volumes of water are withdrawn from ground water and surface water resources to be used in the hydraulic fracturing process.
- Potential Impacts on Drinking Water Resources
- Change in the quantity of water available for drinking
- Change in drinking water quality

Stage 2: Chemical Mixing

- Once delivered to the well site, the acquired water is combined with chemical additives and proppant to make the hydraulic fracturing fluid.
- Potential Impacts on Drinking Water Resources
- Release to surface and ground water through on-site spills and/or leaks

Stage 3: Well Injection

- Pressurized hydraulic fracturing fluid is injected into the well, creating cracks in the geological formation that allow oil or gas to escape through the well to be collected at the surface.
- Potential Impacts on Drinking Water Resources
- Release of hydraulic fracturing fluids to ground water due to inadequate well construction or operation
- Movement of hydraulic fracturing fluids from the target formation to drinking water aquifers through local man-made or natural features (e.g., abandoned wells and existing faults)
- Movement into drinking water aquifers of natural substances found underground, such as metals or radioactive materials, which are mobilized during hydraulic fracturing activities

Stage 4: Flowback and Produced Water (Hydraulic Fracturing Wastewaters)

- When pressure in the well is released, hydraulic fracturing fluid, formation water, and natural gas begin to flow back up the well. This combination of fluids, containing hydraulic fracturing chemical additives and naturally occurring substances, must be stored on-site—typically in tanks or pits—before treatment, recycling, or disposal.
- Potential Impacts on Drinking Water Resources
- Release to surface or ground water through spills or leakage from on-site storage

Stage 5: Wastewater Treatment and Waste Disposal

- Wastewater is dealt with in one of several ways, including but not limited to: disposal by underground injection, treatment followed by disposal to surface water bodies, or recycling (with or without treatment) for use in future hydraulic fracturing operations.
- Potential Impacts on Drinking Water Resources
- Contaminants reaching drinking water due to surface water discharge and inadequate treatment of wastewater.
- Byproducts formed at drinking water treatment facilities by reaction of hydraulic fracturing contaminants with disinfectants. (epa.gov)

"Mr. Fields, can you tell me the reason for your well-known aversion to water?"

W. C. Fields replied "Never touch the stuff. Fish fornicate in it."

In June of 2015, "Congress urged the U.S. Environmental Protection Agency (EPA) to study the relationship between hydraulic fracturing and drinking water. This report synthesizes available scientific literature and data to assess the potential for hydraulic fracturing for oil and gas to change the quality or quantity of drinking water resources, and identifies factors affecting the frequency or severity of any potential changes. This report can be used by federal, tribal, state, and local officials; industry; and the public to better understand and address any vulnerabilities of drinking water resources to hydraulic fracturing activities..." (full report: https://www.epa.gov/sites/production/files/2015-07/documents/hf_es_erd_jun2015.pdf)

Now we have identified a host of wildly toxic chemicals attacking our drinking water from an unlikely source: petrochemical production! We will explore methods of protecting our personal drinking water in a later chapter.

In 2016, "A lawsuit against the EPA could force new, national regulations of the way oil & gas producers dispose of waste. Environmental groups filed suit against the agency, saying the government has failed to adequately regulate disposal of liquid and solid waste generated in the patch. Adam Kron, a lawyer for one of the plaintiffs, says the rules 'are almost 30 years overdue.' Kron, the senior attorney for a group called the Environmental Integrity Project, says it's a 'more waste-intensive industry than ever before.' The lawsuit asks the court to set strict deadlines for the EPA to adopt updated rules." (http://www.newsfromtheoilpatch.com)

FRACKING AND WATER SCARCITY

Water cleanliness and availability has clearly taken a back seat to the concerns of energy production, in the form of hydrofracking. A fracking job can use 140,000 to 150,000 gallons of water per day.

The oil and gas industries enjoy exemptions or outright exclusions for hydraulic fracturing under United States federal law from certain sections of a number of the major federal environmental laws. "These laws range from protecting clean water and air, to preventing the release of toxic substances and chemicals into the environment: the Clean Air Act, Clean Water Act, Safe Drinking Water Act, National Environmental Policy Act, Resource Conservation and Recovery Act, Emergency Planning and Community Right-to-Know Act, and the Comprehensive Environmental Response, Compensation, and Liability Act, commonly known as Superfund."

A 2011 EPA report estimated that 70 to 140 billion gallons of water are used to fracture 35,000 wells in the United States each year — approximately the annual water consumption of 40 to 80 cities each with a population of 50,000, according to Earthworks.

Hydraulically fractured shale regions are outlined in black and overlaid onto a map of U.S. river basins coded by water risk, according to the World Resources Institute's Aqueduct tool. In the following map, river basins colored light yellow have low water stress; basins in dark red have extremely high stress. Almost half of fracked wells in the U.S. are in river basins with high or extremely high risk of water stress.

A recent study by the US Drought Monitor noted that 58 percent of California is experiencing "exceptional drought," which is the most serious category on the agency's five-level scale. A fracking job can require as much as 140,000 to 150,000 gallons of water per day, and this water has won out over agriculture, industrial, or personal use.

Our expertise in our world of drinking water now extends into the realm of controversial production methods of energy production from gas and oil and its possible effects on our fragile drinking water quality and quantity.

Right now: "Switzerland's Linthal hydropower plant produces as much power as a nuclear plant, using nothing but the energy of gravity. It's the world's biggest pumped-storage facility, which means that it works as a kind of giant battery, using water to store electricity in the form of potential energy.

"A pumped storage plant is just what it sounds like. It uses two reservoirs, each at different heights. When power is needed, it runs from the higher reservoir to the lower, passing through turbines in the way, which spin and generate electricity. At night, or at other times of low demand, excess power from the grid is used to reverse the turbines. They become pumps, which pump the water back up into the upper reservoir, effectively storing that surplus electricity for future use. (Requires two mountains, lakes, and a way to bore a hole in the earth. GE is planning more of them.)

(Image from herrenknecht.com)

"The Linthal plant is remarkable mostly because of scale. It uses two mountain lakes 2,000 vertical feet apart, connected by a man-made tunnel. Water runs between Lake Mutt to Lake Limmern, a dammed valley below. Limmern holds 23 billion gallons of water and uses new variable-speed motor generators from General Electric, which improve on fixed-speed designs because their speed can be tailored to suit the amount of power available. Thanks to these motors, the efficiency of the plant is around 80%—that is, just 20% of the generated power is used in pumping the water back up to the top lake..." (fastcoexist.com video: https//youtu.be/5zCf2TXRgpl/)

This amazing Swiss engineering marvel of "free" power production is available now, but we are not using it here in the US!

WATERFICTION: Oil and gas companies are heavily regulated in their fracking operations. Companies are regulated as to where they attain their water for fracking processes.

WATERFACT: There are many exemptions for hydraulic fracturing under United States federal law: the oil and gas industries are exempt or excluded from certain sections of a number of the major federal environmental laws. These laws range from protecting clean water and air, to preventing the release of toxic substances and chemicals into the environment.

"Despite the widespread use of the practice, and the risks hydraulic fracturing poses to human health and safe drinking water supplies, the U.S. Environmental Protection Agency ("EPA") does not regulate the injection of fracturing fluids under the Safe Drinking Water Act. The oil and gas industry is the only industry in America that is allowed by EPA to inject known hazardous materials — unchecked — directly into or adjacent to underground drinking water supplies..." (See more at https://www.earthworksaction.org)

Now that we have identified the offending chemicals that fracking may be introducing into our water, we will take a plunge into the dark waters of lead in our personal drinking water.

Chapter

6

WATER, LEADED and RADIOACTIVE

Lead is definitely mentioned as a regulated toxin on the hit list of EPA, but it deserves our special attention, because the health consequences of exposure are considerable.

World Health Organization (WHO) reports that lead poising can damage nervous and reproductive systems, the kidneys, and cause anemia and high blood pressure. Lead accumulates in the bones and is of particular harm to developing brains of fetuses and young children and pregnant women.

We erroneously believe that the possibilities of our being affected by this dire toxin is remote, but it is a fragile balance as to whether or not we are "lead free." Nearly all homes built prior to 1980 have lead solder joints. Note that, since the Safe Drinking Water Act Amendments of 1986, the use of lead-containing solders in potable water systems has effectively been banned nationwide.

There is no mandate to replace it. The major impact of the Act has been on solder containing 50% tin and 50% lead (50-50), until then the most widely used solder for drinking water systems.

As stated above, lead in our drinking water has become a primary concern because of the severity of its effects on the human body. It is also frighteningly common in our piping. Lead was banned from paint in 1978. It is reported that much of the water infrastructure throughout the country have some lead piping. Lead service lines, also known as branches, connect the water lines in the street to many of our homes and businesses. Roughly 10 million American homes and buildings receive water from service lines that are at least partially lead, according to the Environmental Protection Agency. Service Lead ones are mostly found in the Midwest and Northeast. (https://www2.usgs.gov/blogs/features/usgs_top_story/getting-the-dirt-on-soil/)

There is the 1991 USEPA "lead and copper rule" (LCR), regulating water at the tap, requiring the regular testing of water inside older homes. LCR is in effect today.

From epa.gov:

"The treatment technique for the rule requires systems to monitor drinking water at consumer taps. If lead concentrations exceed an action level of 15 ppb or copper concentrations exceed an action level of 1.3 ppm in more than 10% of customer taps sampled, the system must undertake a number of additional actions to control corrosion. If the action level is exceeded, the system must also inform the public about steps they should take to protect their health and may have to replace lead service lines under their control. While the LCR applies to water utilities, the Reduction of Lead in Drinking Water Act sets standards for pipe, plumbing fittings, fixtures, solder and flux." Very reassuring.

Water and Waste Digest reports that more than 5,000 water systems violate the Lead & Copper Rule, and more than 18 million Americans received drinking water from systems with lead violations in 2015, according to a Natural Resources Defense Council (NRDC) report. According to NRDC scientists and health experts, the problem could be significantly more pervasive because many more water systems known to have such violations — including that in Flint, Michigan — do not show up as having lead violations in the government database designed to track such problems.

"Americans take it for granted that the water flowing from their home taps is clean and safe, but all too often that assumption is wrong," said Erik Olson, health program director for NRDC. "Shoddy data collection, lax enforcement of the law and cities gaming the system have created a potent brew of lead violations and unsafe drinking water from the water supplies used by millions of people across the nation."

"What's In Your Water: Flint and Beyond" documents lead in drinking water issues across the U.S. The peer-reviewed report offers explores the issues that contributed to widespread lead contamination in Flint, mapping EPA violations for the federal Lead and Copper Rule, and documenting the lack of enforcement against those violations. NRDC's analysis and accompanying digital maps expose the scope of lead-related issues in drinking water systems across the U.S. The report found that more than 18 million people were served by 5,363 community water systems that violated the Lead and Copper Rule. These violations included failure to treat to reduce lead levels, monitor for lead, and report test results to citizens or the government.

Not every person served by these systems is known to have excessive lead in his or her water, because only a small percentage of homes were tested, and lead levels can vary from home to home. However, according to industry estimates, 15 million to 22 million Americans are served drinking water through lead service line (the pipe connecting a residence to the water main) that can release lead into tap water. (http://www.wwdmag.com/contaminants/nrdc-report-documents-widespread-leadviolations?eid=216791542&bid=1457560)

"A whopping nine out of 10 of these water rule violations never faced any formal enforcement. In fact, states and EPA sought penalties against only 3% of Lead Rule violators. That's inexcusable. The message sent to water suppliers that knowingly violate the law is clear: There is no cop on the beat," Olson said.

In a 2016 report conducted using data from the EPA's Safe Drinking Water Information System (SDWIS) database, over 6 million people and 2,000 water systems have excessive lead levels in the drinking water over a 4 year span.

It is a federal law but it is enforced on the local level. This is where the finger pointing begins.

If there is a break in a branch that is lead, the utility will replace it with non-lead, but the homeowner is obligated to replace the line from the curb to the house.

Water and Wastes Digest reports that "there are about 6.1 million lead service lines nationwide. If the average cost of replacing each one is $5000, then the collective cost could easily top $30 billion, according to American Water Works Association. This is in addition to the $1 trillion needed over 25 years to repair and expand buried drinking water mains."

Despite the bewildering consequences of lead poising, there is no plan to replace these pipes. Corrosion control by means of chemicals that coat the inside of the pipes is the remedy preferred, instead of digging them up and replacing them, but they can and do fail if the water chemistry changes enough.

One of the common additives to control corrosion of the lead pipes is phosphoric acid, but there is the possible consequence of the phosphorous contaminating lakes, waterways, and watersheds.

There was a historic incident in the U.S. town of Flint, Michigan. The report reads more like a mystery novel than a water report. It is an example of complete failure of government controls.

LESSONS FROM FLINT, MICHIGAN

In April 2014, Flint had been buying their municipal water from Detroit, Michigan for millions of dollars that they could apparently no longer afford. A decision was made there to shut off the valve to Detroit, save the money, and to open the valve and begin using the water from Flint River. The result was catastrophic and led to federal prosecutions.

The NY Times chronology:
http://www.nytimes.com/interactive/2016/01/21/us/flint-lead-water-timeline.html

The minimization of corrosion in our water pipes is high science. Phosphate in the form of bimetallic phosphates, polyphosphates, orthophosphates, and glassy phosphates are often used to control corrosive conditions within our pipes.

How does lead get into my tap water?

> Measures taken during the last two decades have greatly reduced exposures to lead in tap water. These measures include actions taken under the requirements of the 1986 and 1996 amendments to the Safe Drinking Water Act.

> Even so, lead still can be found in some metal water taps, interior water pipes, or pipes connecting a house to the main water pipe in the street. Lead found in tap water usually comes from the corrosion of older fixtures or from the solder that connects pipes. When water sits in leaded pipes for several hours, lead can leach into the water supply.

How do I know if my tap water is contaminated with lead?

> The only way to know whether your tap water contains lead is to have it tested. You cannot see, taste, or smell lead in drinking water. Therefore, you must ask your water provider whether your water has lead in it. For homes served by public water systems, data on lead in tap water may be available on the Internet from your local water authority. If your water provider does not post this information, you should call and find out.

Does a high lead level in my tap water cause health effects?

> High levels of lead in tap water can cause health effects if the lead in the water enters the bloodstream and causes an elevated blood lead level.

> Most studies show that exposure to lead-contaminated water alone would not be likely to elevate blood lead

levels in most adults, even exposure to water with a lead content close to the EPA action level for lead of 15 parts per billion (ppb). Risk will vary, however, depending on the individual, the circumstances, and the amount of water consumed. For example, infants who drink formula prepared with lead-contaminated water may be at a higher risk because of the large volume of water they consume relative to their body size.

What can I do to reduce or eliminate lead in my tap water?

If your tap water contains lead at levels exceeding EPA's action level of 15 ppb, you should take action to minimize your exposure to the lead in the water.

You should begin by asking your water authority these questions:

1. Does my water have lead in it above EPA's action level of 15 parts per billion (ppb)?
   If the answer is no, no action is needed.
   If the answer is yes, also ask the next question:

2. Does the service pipe at the street (header pipe) have lead in it?
   This information is very important. It determines which of the next two actions (A or B) you should follow to protect your household's health.
   A) If the pipe in the street (header pipe) DOES NOT have lead, the lead in your tap water may be coming from fixtures, pipes, or elsewhere inside your home.
      Until you eliminate the source, you should take the following steps any time you wish to use tap water for drinking or cooking, especially when the water has been off and sitting in the pipes for more than 6 hours:
      a. Before using any tap water for drinking or cooking, flush your water system by running the kitchen tap (or any other tap you take drinking or cooking water from) on COLD for 1–2 minutes;

     b. Then, fill a clean container(s) with water from this tap. This water will be suitable for drinking, cooking, preparation of baby formula, or other consumption. To conserve water, collect multiple containers of water at once (after you have fully flushed the water from the tap as described).

B) If the pipe at the street (header pipe) DOES contain lead, lead in the tap water may be coming from that pipe or connected pipes (it may also be coming from sources inside your home). Until the lead source is eliminated, you should take the following steps any time you wish to use tap water for drinking or cooking, especially when the water has been off and sitting in the pipes for more than 6 hours. Please note that additional flushing is necessary:

     a. Before using any tap water for drinking or cooking, run high-volume taps (such as your shower) on COLD for 5 minutes or more;

     b. Then, run the kitchen tap on COLD for 1–2 additional minutes;

     c. Fill a clean container(s) with water from this tap. This water will be suitable for drinking, cooking, preparation of baby formula, or other consumption. To conserve water, collect multiple containers of water at once (after you have fully flushed the water from the tap as described).

3. In all situations, drink or cook only with water that comes out of the tap cold. Water that comes out of the tap warm or hot can contain much higher levels of lead. Boiling this water will NOT reduce the amount of lead in your water.

4. You can also reduce or eliminate your exposure to lead in drinking water by consuming only bottled water or water from a filtration system that has been certified by an independent testing organization to reduce or eliminate lead....

5. Children and pregnant women are especially vulnerable to the effects of lead exposure. Therefore, for homes with children or pregnant

women and with water lead levels exceeding EPA's action level of 15 ppb, CDC recommends using bottled water or water from a filtration system that has been certified by an independent testing organization to reduce or eliminate lead for cooking, drinking, and baby formula preparation. Because most bottled water does not contain fluoride, a fluoride supplement may be necessary.

Also, some bottled waters have not been tested and may not be appropriate for consumption. Contact independent testing organizations that certify bottled water....

6. Make sure that repairs to copper pipes do not use lead solder. Advice for lead safe water practices after plumbing work in housing with lead water lines or lead solder.

   These practices include
   1. Testing water after plumbing work in older housing. Please contact your state lead program for information about water testing in your area.
   2. Inspecting the aerator on the end of the faucet and removing any debris such as metal particles.
   3. Flushing water lines before using the water for drinking or cooking.

If you own your home, you may also consider full replacement of lead water lines by removing the private lines running from the water meter into your home. This precaution has not been adequately studied, however, because the data available to CDC included too few homes having had full replacement of lead water lines. Contact your water authority for information about replacing water service lines.

If my water has high lead levels, is it safe to take a bath or shower?

Yes. Bathing and showering should be safe for you and your children, even if the water contains lead over EPA's action level. Human skin does not absorb lead in water. (https://www.cdc.gov/nceh/lead/tips/water.htm)

Drinking water delivered through lead pipes or pipes joined with lead solder may contain lead. Much of the lead in global commerce is now obtained from recycling.

Young children are particularly vulnerable to the toxic effects of lead and can suffer profound and permanent adverse health effects, particularly affecting the development of the brain and nervous system. Lead also causes long-term harm in adults, including increased risk of high blood pressure and kidney damage. Exposure of pregnant women to high levels of lead can cause miscarriage, stillbirth, premature birth and low birth weight, as well as minor malformations.

Sources and routes of exposure:

People can become exposed to lead through occupational and environmental sources. This mainly results from:

- inhalation of lead particles generated by burning materials containing lead, e.g. during smelting, informal recycling, stripping leaded paint and using leaded gasoline; and
- ingestion of lead-contaminated dust, water (from leaded pipes), food (from lead-glazed or lead-soldered containers).

Health effects of lead poisoning on children: Lead has had serious consequences for the health of children. At high levels of exposure, lead attacks the brain and central nervous system to cause coma, convulsions and even death. Children who survive severe lead poisoning may be left with mental retardation and behavioral disruption. At lower levels of exposure that cause no obvious symptoms, and that previously were considered safe, lead is now known to produce a spectrum of injury across multiple body systems. In particular lead affects children's brain development resulting in reduced intelligence quotient (IQ), behavioral changes such as shortening of attention span and increased antisocial behavior, and reduced educational attainment. Lead exposure also causes anemia, hypertension, renal impairment, immunotoxicity and toxicity to the reproductive organs. The neurological and behavioral effects of lead are believed to be irreversible.

There is no known safe blood lead concentration. But it is known that, as lead exposure increases, the range and severity of symptoms and effects also increases. Even blood lead concentrations as low as 5 µg/dl, once thought to be a 'safe level', may result in decreased intelligence in children, behavioral difficulties and learning problems.

Encouragingly, the successful phasing out of leaded gasoline in most countries has resulted in a significant decline in population-level blood lead concentrations. There are now only six countries that continue to use leaded fuel.

WHO response

WHO has identified lead as one of ten chemicals of major public health concern, needing action by Member States to protect the health of workers, children and women of reproductive age.

WHO has made available through its website a range of information on lead, including information for policy makers, technical guidance and advocacy materials.

WHO is currently developing guidelines on the prevention and management of lead poisoning, which will provide policy-makers, public health authorities and health professionals with evidence-based guidance on the measures that they can take to protect the health of children and adults from lead exposure.

Since leaded paint is a continuing source of exposure in many countries, WHO has joined with the United Nations Environment Program to form the Global Alliance to Eliminate Lead Paint. This is a cooperative initiative to focus and catalyze efforts to achieve international goals to prevent children's exposure to lead from leaded paints and to minimize occupational exposures to such paint. Its broad objective is to promote a phase-out of the manufacture and sale of paints containing lead and eventually eliminate the risks that such paints pose.

The Global Alliance to Eliminate Lead Paint is an important means of contributing to the implementation of paragraph 57 of the Plan of

Implementation of the World Summit on Sustainable Development and to resolution II/4B of the Strategic Approach to International Chemicals Management (SAICM), which both concern the phasing of lead paint." (http://www.who.int/mediacentre/factsheets/fs379/en/)

This information applies to most situations and to a large majority of the population, but individual circumstances may vary. Some situations, such as cases involving highly corrosive water, may require additional recommendations or more stringent actions. Your local water authority is always your first source for testing and identifying lead contamination in your tap water. Many public water authorities have websites that include data on drinking water quality, including results of lead testing..." (https://www.cdc.gov/nceh/lead/tips/water.htm)

Wired Magazine reports the leaded water crisis in Flint is just the beginning of an epidemic:

> In early 2003 an Environmental Protection Agency subcontractor called Cadmus Group was looking into a singular problem: Homes all over Washington, DC, were springing pinhole leaks in their water pipes. So Cadmus hired a young environmental engineer at Virginia Tech named Marc Edwards as a consultant.
>
> The leaks seemed confined to residential copper. PVC pipes and municipal lines weren't leaking. That made Edwards think that the problem was in the city water supply. In the US, municipal drinking water is protected by the Safe Drinking Water Act, which compels utilities to monitor things like microorganisms and the disinfectants used to subdue them. In 1998 the EPA tightened its standards on disinfectants, many of which can have their own toxic byproducts. One of the worst offenders is a classic: chlorine. Its main replacement, a chemical called chloramine (really just a mix of chlorine and ammonia), has lower levels of carcinogenic breakdown products, but it also makes the water corrosive—enough to eat through metal.

It turned out that the District of Columbia's Water and Sewer Authority had in fact swapped chlorine for chloramine in 2000. But when Edwards went into homes to check the damage, he discovered something even scarier than leaks. The corrosive water was burning through service lines and solders—and those contained lead. The water was even pitting the lead-infused brass in water meters and faucets... (https://www.wired.com/2016/06/flint-water-marc-edwards/)

REMOVAL OF LEAD FROM CONTAMINATED WATER

According to a group of professors from Temple University and Philadelphia University, over the past 25 years, about 750,000 sites with potential contamination have been reported to federal or state authorities. Heavy metals are the largest class of contaminants and also the most difficult to treat. Lead pollution impacts all the systems of the human body. Many of the methods utilized to remove lead from wastewater have shortcomings:

Essentially all industrial processes generate by-products that become waste materials. These waste materials have the potential of contaminating the environment. Heavy metals, solvents organic compounds, and petroleum products account for most of the contaminants. The adverse impact of heavy metals, especially lead, on the environment and living organisms have been well documented by many researchers. Living organisms need trace amounts of some heavy metals, including cobalt, copper, iron, manganese, molybdenum, vanadium, strontium, and zinc. However, there is a limit beyond which it can be damaging to the organism. Non-essential heavy metals that are harmful to living organisms and have been encountered in both underground water and surface water systems are cadmium, chromium, mercury, lead, arsenic, and antimony.

Heavy metals have been used in a variety of ways for many centuries. For the past three centuries, the production of heavy metals such as lead, copper, and zinc has increased exponentially. Plumbing and insect control (as lead arsenate in apple orchards) are a couple of common examples of lead application. Exposure to heavy metals leads to developmental retardation, various cancers, kidney damage, and even death in some instances. Exposure to high levels of lead has also been associated with the development of autoimmunity....

Heavy metals are present in more than half of Department of Defense (DOD), superfund, Department of Energy (DOE) and Resource Conservation and Recovery Act (RCRA) sites. The primary heavy metals of concern are arsenic, lead, cadmium, chromium, and mercury. Various forms of these metals may enter the environment from sources including abandoned dumping sites, wastes from metal plating and metal smelting, by-products from refining operations, and from manufacturing of computer components. According to EPA there are over 200,000 contaminated sites in the United States alone that requires remediation. The estimated expense for this massive undertaking is at least $750 billion and can reach $1 trillion. Lead is one of the most problematic heavy metals. Lead is dangerous to human health and the ecosystem because: a) Lead is in elemental form, and hence cannot be degraded or transformed into a less dangerous material, b) Lead is highly harmful to living organisms even in very low concentration, c) Lead contamination is already widespread in the ecosystem. Lead exposure in humans can have severe neurological and physiological repercussions....

CONCLUSIONS: The removal mechanism of lead from contaminated water varies based on the pH of the solution. At high pH the removal is mainly precipitation of heavy metal to the surface of the barrier materials. The adsorption is removal mechanism as the pH level drops below 9 while the pH is lower than 6, the removal process is the ion exchange. Removal of heavy metals such as lead from industrial processes can be grouped in several known techniques. Some of the most effective methods to remove lead from contaminated waters are precipitation stabilization, ion exchange and adsorption. Investigation of AAM (Alkali Ash Material) in the past 3 years has demonstrated that fly ash can be transformed into an effective sorbent for heavy metals. AAM has the ability to remove heavy metals such as Pb from contaminated solution. 1000 ppm of Pb solution was reduced to about 0.6 ppm after passing through the optimized Controlled Permeability AAM contamination barrier. The process has been successful with class F fly ash from many sources. Additional work in this area is required.

(Brooks, R. M., Bahadory, M., Tovia, F., & Rostami, H. (2010). "Removal of lead from contaminated water." *International journal of soil, sediment and water*, 3(2), 14.)

We will discuss additional options to control our personal water quality in a later chapter.

"Life in us is like the water in a river."

- Henry David Thoreau

WATERFICTION: Boiling my water will render it lead free.

WATERFACT: Some of the water evaporates during the boiling process, and the lead concentration of the water can actually increase slightly as the water is boiled. If it is not possible or cost-effective to remove the lead source, (i.e. lead pipes) flushing the water system before using the water for drinking or cooking may be an option. In all situations, drink or cook only with water that comes out of the tap cold. Water that comes out of the tap warm or hot can contain much higher levels of lead. Boiling this water will NOT reduce the amount of lead in your water. Bathing and showering should be safe for you and your children, even if the water contains lead over EPA's action level. Human skin does not absorb lead in water.

Chapter

7

THE TWISTED SISTERS, FLUORIDE AND CHLORINE

Voluntary additives to our fragile municipal water systems are rare. Chlorine and fluoride are center stage in our saga, and both have dark histories and known human toxicities. These rogue siblings roam our reported million miles of pipes — and were actually invited!

We will discuss chlorine first, as she has the redeeming quality of being a cheap way to somewhat contain things like typhoid that may grow there.

Buckle up, wear rubber gloves, and no running.

WATER COMING CLEAN, CHLORINE

What happens when we get too much of a good thing? That is the case when chlorine additives are used to purify our drinking water. We will discuss the chemistry of, history of, benefits of, and the dark side of this familiar chemical, chlorine. It makes us think of bright and white laundry, billowing in the breeze on a summer's day.

Add it to our drinking water and we get confused ... literally!

We have identified the usual suspect chemicals in the crime of toxifying our drinking water. These chemical criminals infiltrate and desecrate our drinking water by way of physical failures: in the case of lead and copper, leached from ancient pipes; breaks in water mains; pesticide runoff; industrial spills and dumping; natural geological process; chemical processes; mismanaged sewage; failures within treatment facilities; and a plethora of other obscure sources. Have we addressed every imagined and imaginable problem that a simple glass or bottle of water could possess, or be possessed by? Hardly. This is our daily game of water roulette personified.

Now we will continue our safari into the world of what is intentionally added to our municipal drinking water systems in the name of protecting us — welcome to chlorineland. Everyone stay together, turn off those cell phones, and for goodness's sake no running or gum chewing.

Chlorine (Cl_2) is also known as hypochlorite. It the common element we hear of in association with keeping our water clean and pure. The first appearance is in the late 1800's in Europe, and in 1908 in the U.S., at Boonton Reservoir on the Rockaway River, which supplied Jersey City, New Jersey.

This highly toxic chemical acts to kill bacteria. Chlorinating water acts to kill certain bacteria and other microbes in our water system as chlorine is highly toxic. In particular, chlorination is used to prevent the spread of waterborne diseases such as cholera and typhoid. It is used to combat microbial contamination but it can mix with certain organic matter and create Disinfection By-Products (DPBs) which are also identified as carcinogenic trihalomethanes. A reported 90% of the US population drinks chlorinated water, which may contain many of those DPSs.

But wait.

Chlorine in small doses is known to cause coughing and sneezing, running nose, and red eyes, and can be fatal in large doses. Chlorine gas was actually used in WWI by Germany as a weapon! It killed and crippled many during that war as a result of throat and lung damage.

Overview:

Chlorine ranks among the top 10 chemicals produced in the United States. In 1992, about 10.5 billion kilograms (23 billion pounds) of the element were produced in the United States. Chlorine, in one form or another, is added to most swimming pools, spas, and public water supplies because it kills bacteria that cause disease. Many people also use chlorine to bleach their clothes. Large paper and pulp mills use chlorine to bleach their products.

Chlorine is a greenish-yellow poisonous gas. It was discovered in 1774 by Swedish chemist Carl Wilhelm Scheele (1742-86). Scheele knew that chlorine was a new element, but thought it contained oxygen as well.

SYMBOL Cl ATOMIC NUMBER 17 ATOMIC MASS 35.453 FAMILY Group 17 (VIIA)

Halogen:

Chlorine is a member of the halogen family. Halogens are the elements that make up Group 17 (VIIA) of the periodic table, a chart that shows how elements are related to one another. They include fluorine, bromine, iodine, and astatine. Chlorine is highly reactive, ranking only below fluorine in its chemical activity....

Chlorine occurs commonly both in the Earth's crust and in seawater.

The true nature of Scheele's discovery was not completely understood for many years. Some chemists argued that his dephlogisticated marine acid was really a compound of a new element and oxygen. This confusion was finally cleared up in 1807. English chemist Sir Humphry Davy (1778-1829) proved that Scheele's substance was a pure element. He suggested the name chlorine for the element, from the Greek word chloros, meaning "greenish-yellow."

Physical properties:

Chlorine is a dense gas with a density of 3.21 grams per liter. By comparison, the density of air is 1.29 grams per liter. Chlorine changes from a gas into a liquid at a temperature of -34.05°C (-29.29°F) and from a liquid to a solid at -101.00°C (-149.80°F). The gas is soluble (dissolvable) in water. It also reacts chemically with water as it dissolves to form hydrochloric acid (HCl) and hypochlorous acid (HOCl).

Chemical properties:

Chlorine is a very active element. It combines with all elements except the noble gases. The noble gases are the elements that make up Group 18 (VIIIA) of the periodic table. The reaction between chlorine and other elements can often be vigorous. For example, chlorine reacts explosively with hydrogen to form hydrogen chloride:

Chlorine does not burn but, like oxygen, it helps other substances burn. Chlorine is a strong oxidizing agent (a chemical substance that gives up or takes on electrons from another substance).

Occurrence in nature:

Chlorine occurs commonly both in the Earth's crust and in seawater. Its abundance in the earth is about 100 to 300 parts per million. It ranks 20th among the elements in abundance in the earth. Its abundance in seawater is about 2 percent. The most common compound of chlorine in seawater is sodium chloride. Smaller amounts of potassium chloride also occur in seawater.

The most common minerals of chlorine are halite, or rock salt (NaCl), sylvite (KCl), and camallite (KCl MgCl 2). Large amounts of these minerals are mined from underground salt beds that were formed when ancient oceans dried up. Over millions of years, the salts that remained behind were buried underground. They were also compacted (packed together) to form huge salt "domes." A salt dome is a large mass of salt found underground.

Isotopes:

Two naturally occurring isotopes of chlorine exist, chlorine-35 and chlorine-36. Isotopes are two or more forms of an element. Isotopes differ from each other according to their mass number. The number written to the right of the element's name is the mass number. The mass number represents the number of protons plus neutrons in the nucleus of an atom of the element. The number of protons determines the element, but the number of neutrons in the atom of any one element can vary. Each variation is an isotope.

Seven radioactive isotopes of chlorine are also known. A radioactive isotope is one that breaks apart and gives off some form of radiation. Radioactive isotopes are produced when very small particles are fired at atoms. These particles stick in the atoms and make them radioactive.

One radioactive isotope of chlorine is used in research. That isotope is chlorine-36. This isotope is used because compounds of chlorine occur so commonly in everyday life. The behavior of these compounds can be studied if chlorine-36 is used as a tracer. A tracer is an isotope whose presence in a material can be traced (followed) easily....

Extraction:

Chlorine is produced by passing an electric current through a water solution of sodium chloride or through molten (melted) sodium chloride. This process is one of the most important commercial processes in industry. The products formed include two of the most widely used materials: sodium hydroxide (NaOH) and chlorine (Cl 2). With a water solution, the reaction that occurs is:

Hydrogen gas (H 2) is also formed in the reaction.

Uses and compounds:

Chlorine is widely used throughout the world to purify water. In the United States, only about 6 percent of the chlorine manufactured is used in water purification. About three times as much is used in the paper and pulp industry as a bleach. The most important use of chlorine is to make other chemicals. For example, chlorine can be combined with ethene, or ethylene, gas (C 2) H 2), to make ethylene dichloride (C 2)H 2)Cl 2): Large amounts of chlorine minerals are mined from underground salt beds that were formed when ancient oceans dried up.

About one-third of the chlorine produced in the United States goes to making ethylene dichloride. About 90 percent of ethylene dichloride goes to the manufacture of polyvinyl chloride (PVC). PVC is used to make piping, tubing, flooring, siding, film, coatings, and many other products. Ethylene dichloride has become one of the most popular products in American industry. About 4.5 billion kilograms (10 billion pounds) of the material are made each year.

Are we getting poisoned?

One of the most troubling uses of chlorine has been in making pesticides. A pesticide is a chemical used to kill pests. Pesticides have special names depending on the kind of pests they are designed to kill. Insecticides kill insects, rodenticides kill rodents (rats and mice), fungicides kill fungi, and nematicides kill worms.

Certain chlorine compounds have become very popular as pesticides. These compounds are called chlorinated hydrocarbons. They contain carbon, hydrogen, and chlorine.

Probably the most famous chlorinated hydrocarbon is dichlorodiphenyltrichloroethane, or DDT. DDT was first prepared in 1873, but was not used as a pesticide until World War II (1939-45). Public health officials were at first delighted to learn that DDT kills disease-carrying insects very efficiently. There was great hope that DDT could be used to wipe out certain diseases in some parts of the world.

Farmers were also excited about DDT. They found it could kill many of the pests that attacked crops. By the end of the 1950s, many farmers were spraying huge amounts of DDT on their land to get rid of pests.

But problems began to appear. Many fish and birds in sprayed areas began to die or become deformed. Soon, these problems were traced to the use of DDT. The fish and birds ate insects that had been sprayed with DDT or drank water that contained DDT. It had a toxic effect on the fish and birds, just as it did on insects. Bird populations declined drastically as DDT caused eggs to be so thin-shelled that young birds did not survive.

Eventually, many governments began to ban the use of DDT. Since 1973, the United States has not allowed the compound to be used. It is still used in other nations of the world, however. These nations feel that the benefits of using DDT outweigh the harm it may cause. They feel that DDT can save lives by killing disease-causing pests. They know they can increase their food supplies by using DDT on crops.

DDT is not the only chlorinated hydrocarbon used as a pesticide. Other compounds in this class include dieldrin, aldrin, heptachlor, and chlordan. The use of these compounds has also been banned or restricted in the United States. The U.S. government has decided the harm they cause to the environment is more important than the benefits they provide to farmers and other users.

Another compound made using chlorine is propylene oxide (CH 3 CH0CH 2). There is no chlorine in propylene oxide, but chlorine is used in the process by which the compound is made. Propylene oxide is used to make a group of plastics known as polyesters. Polyesters are found in a wide range of materials, including car and boat bodies, bowling balls, fabrics for clothing, and rugs.

At one time, a large amount of chlorine was used to make a group of compounds known as chlorofluorocarbons (CFCs). CFCs are a family of chemical compounds containing carbon, fluorine, and chlorine. CFCs were once used in a wide variety of applications, such as air conditioning and refrigeration, aerosol spray products, and cleaning materials. They are now known to have serious environmental effects and have been banned from use in the United States and many other countries in the world.

The reason for this ban is the damage caused by CFCs on the Earth's ozone layer. Ozone (O 3) is a form of oxygen that filters out harmful radiation from the sun. When CFCs escape into the atmosphere, they attack and destroy ozone molecules. They reduce the protection against radiation provided by ozone.

Health effects

WARTIME CHLORINE:

Chlorine gas is extremely toxic and in larger doses, chlorine can be fatal. In fact, chlorine gas was used during World War I (1914-18) by the German army as a weapon. Thousands of soldiers were killed or seriously wounded by breathing it. Those who survived gas attacks often were crippled for life. They were unable to breathe normally as a result of the damage to their throats and lungs.

In plants, chlorine is regarded as a micronutrient, which is a substance needed in very small amounts to maintain good health. Leaves turn yellow and die when plants get too little chlorine from the soil.

Chlorine is produced by passing an electric current through a water solution of sodium chloride or through molten (melted) sodium chloride.

Compounds of chlorine are important in maintaining good health in humans and animals. The average human body contains about 95 grams (about 3.5 ounces) of chlorine. Hydrochloric acid (HCl) in the stomach, for example, helps in the digestion of foods. Sodium chloride ($NaCl$) and potassium chloride (KCl) play an important role in the way nerve messages are sent throughout the body. Because humans eat so much salt, a lack of chlorine compounds is seldom a health problem...

(http://www.chemistryexplained.com/elements/A-C/Chlorine.html)

Safe Water Drinking Act:

In 1974, Congress passed the Safe Drinking Water Act. This law requires the EPA to determine the level of residual disinfectants in drinking water at which no adverse health effects are likely to occur. These non-enforceable health goals, based solely on possible health risks and exposure over a lifetime, with an adequate margin of safety, are called maximum residual disinfectant level goals (MRDLG). Contaminants are any physical, chemical, biological, or radiological substances or matter in water. EPA sets MRDLGs based on the best available science to prevent potential health problems.

Disinfectant	*MRDLG*	*MRDL*
Chloramine	4 milligrams per liter (mg/L)	4.0 mg/L
	or 4 parts per million (ppm)	or 4 ppm as an annual average
Chlorine	4 mg/L or 4 ppm	4.0 mg/L
		or 4 ppm as an annual average
Chlorine Dioxide	0.8 mg/L	0.8 mg/L or 800 ppb
	or 800 parts per billion (ppb)	

MRDLs are set as close to the health goals as possible, considering cost, benefits, and the ability of public water systems to detect and remove contaminants using suitable treatment technologies. In this case, the MRDL equals the MRDLG, because analytical methods or treatment technology do not pose any limitation. States may set more stringent drinking water MRDLGs and MRDLs for disinfectants than EPA.

> According to the U.S. Environmental Protection Agency (EPA), chlorine levels of four parts per million or below in drinking water—whether from a private well or municipal reservoir—are acceptable from a human health standpoint.

It was so effective at destroying potentially harmful bacteria and viruses that the practice soon became common practice. Today some 98 percent of water treatment facilities in the U.S. use some form of chlorine to clean drinking water supplies. The American Water Works Association (AWWA), a trade group representing water utilities across the country, credits the presence of chlorine in drinking water with a 50 percent increase in life expectancy for Americans over the last century. Indeed, some consider the chlorination of drinking water to be one of history's greatest public health achievements.

But others aren't so sure that any chlorine in drinking water should be considered safe. Opponents of chlorination point to studies linking repeated exposure to trace amounts of chlorine in water with higher incidences of bladder, rectal and breast cancers. The problem lies in chlorine's ability to interact with organic compounds in fresh water to create trihalomethanes (THMs), which when ingested can encourage the growth of free radicals that can destroy or damage vital cells in the body. Besides cancer, exposure to THMs has been linked to other health issues including asthma, eczema, heart disease and higher miscarriage and birth defect rates.

Those with their own private wells who are skittish about chlorine have other options for disinfecting their water. One baby step would be to replace chlorine with chloramine, an ammonia derivative that doesn't dissipate into the environment as rapidly as chlorine and has a much lower tendency to interact in bad ways with organic compounds in the water. However, traces of chloramine in the water may not be to everyone's liking either, because it causes rashes after showering in a small percentage of people and can apparently increase lead exposure in older homes as it leaches the heavy metal off old pipes.

Another option, though somewhat costly, would be to purchase a machine to purify the water. Ozonation units, which disinfect by adding ozone molecules to water and leave no residues, start at around $9,000. Another choice would be a UV light treatment machine—at $6,000 or more—which cancels out viruses and bacteria by passing the water through UV light rays. There are more methods of removal covered in Chapter 9.

Perhaps the most sensible and affordable approach is to filter the water at the faucets and taps. Carbon-based tap- or pitcher-mounted filters can work wonders in removing impurities from drinking water. They can even be installed on shower heads for those with sensitive skin... (https://www.scientificamerican.com/article/i-was-wondering-how-toxic-chlorine-is/)

How widespread is the use of chlorine today?

The addition of chlorine in drinking water has been the standard in water treatment in the United States since 1904. Thus, for over 100 years we have trusted and relied on chlorine to purify our water and kill off any waterborne pathogens.

The good News of Chlorine in Drinking water: that chlorine has done a good job in killing off most microorganisms in the water. In fact, the United States has one of the safest water supplies in the world, and I am truly grateful for this. Without chlorine (or some other form of water disinfection treatment), millions of people would die from devastating infections such as cholera, salmonella, and others.

The Bad of News Chlorine in Drinking Water: chlorine treatment does not absolutely ensure that by the time our drinking water comes out of our home faucet it is free of unhealthy microorganisms. It may sit in our pipes for a while, collecting bacteria and such!

Dangerous bacteria such as e-coli and coliform are still found in chlorinated tap water on occasion. When this happens it is primarily due to problems related to the treatment system itself or to the transport of the water to our homes. Thus, relying on chlorine disinfection alone is a false guarantee that the water from your tap is safe to drink. Even minimal exposure to these types of bacteria can cause symptoms similar to the flu, such as headaches, diarrhea, cramps, nausea or vomiting.

Thus, I highly recommend a tap water filter at the point-of-use (your water faucet) to ensure adequate filtration of unhealthy micro-organisms, as well as other many other contaminants, that could end up in your drinking water.

The Ugly Side of Chlorine in Drinking Water:

The ugly side of drinking chlorinated water has only recently been documented. And it has to do with the long-term health effects of chlorine and its disinfection by-products (DBPs).

What the studies have found is that chlorine itself is not the main problem; rather it has to do with what happens when the chlorine mixes with any type of organic matter in the water.

In the 1970s scientists discovered that when chlorine is added to water, it forms Trihalomethanes (THMs), one of which is chloroform. THMs increase the production of free radicals in the body and are highly carcinogenic (cancer causing).

Chlorine and THMS have been linked to various types of cancer, kidney and liver damage, immune system dysfunction, disorders of the nervous system, hardening of the arteries, and birth defects.

Negative Effects of DBPs and Chlorine:

Unfortunately, we are learning the hard way that our attempts to prevent illness by adding chlorine in drinking water has contributed to another problem—the increase of cancer and heart disease. Check out what the experts have to say:

"Cancer risk among people using chlorinated water is as much as 93 percent higher than among those whose water does not contain chlorine," according to the U.S. Council of Environmental Quality:

"One common factor among women with breast cancer is that they all have 50 to 60 percent higher levels of these chlorination by-products (THMs) in their fat tissue than women without breast cancer."

"Long-term drinking of chlorinated water appears to increase a person's risk of developing bladder cancer as much as 80 percent," as documented in a study published in the Journal of the National Cancer Institute. Some 45,000 Americans are diagnosed every year with bladder cancer...

"The drinking of chlorinated water has finally been officially linked to an increased incidence of colon cancer. An epidemiologist at Oak Ridge Associated Universities completed a study of colon cancer victims and non-cancer patients and concluded that the drinking of chlorinated water for 15 years or more was conducive to a high rate of colon cancer," according to Health Freedom News, January/February 1987.

But drinking chlorinated water is only half the problem. Bathing and showering in unfiltered tap water is just as bad as drinking it, according to the Journal of Public Health

and numerous other scientists and doctors.... (http://www.
waterbenefitshealth.com/chlorine-in-drinking-water.html)

A Better Way to Disinfect Water:

Shock chlorination:

Shock chlorination is a process used in many swimming pools, water wells,
springs, and other water sources to reduce the bacterial and algal residue
in the water. Shock chlorination is performed by mixing a large amount
of hypochlorite into the water. The hypochlorite can be in the form of a
powder or a liquid such as chlorine bleach (solution of sodium hypochlorite
in water). Water that is being shock chlorinated should not be swum in or
drunk until the sodium hypochlorite count in the water goes down to three
parts per million (PPM) or less.

Alternative methods for water disinfection:

Ozonation:

Ozonation is used in many European countries and on occasion in Canada
and U.S.A. This alternative is more cost effective but energy intensive.
Ozone is aerated or bubbled through water being bubbled through the
water resulting in the breaking down of parasites, bacteria, and other
harmful organic substances. Unfortunately, ozonation leaves no residual
ozone to continue the disinfection process.

Chlorination remains in the pipes. The advantage of chlorine in comparison
to ozone is that the residual chlorine remains in the water for an extended
period of time.

Chloramination:

Chloramination is also used as an alternative. Disinfection with chloramine
produces less undesirable byproducts than chlorine (gas or hypochlorite).
Chloramine has a half-life longer then chlorine, and remains effective
for longer periods of time, and maintains effective protection against
pathogens. (Chloramine is formed by adding ammonia and chlorine into

drinking water and this forms monochloramine and/or dichloramine.) The organisms Helicobacter pylori and Escherichia coli are effectively disinfected by chloramine and are equally susceptible to the disinfecting effect of chloramine.

Bromination and iodinization

Chlorine is three times more effective against Escherichia coli than an amount of bromine, and six times that of concentrated iodine.

Home filtration:

Filtration may render water safe. Many pathogens are removed by materials in the filter bed. Filtered water must be drank soon after filtration, or residual pathogens may grow. Home filters generally remove 90% of chlorine. Filters must be replaced periodically of the bacteria within the unit may actually grow in the water.

Ultra Violet Radiation

Ultra Violet (UV) treatment leaves minimal residue in the water. In water, UV generates ozone *in situ* and thus has many of the advantages of ozone disinfection above. However, this method alone will not remove toxins from the water.

Reverse Osmosis (RO)

RO is a water purification technology that makes use of a semipermeable membrane for removal of molecules, ions, bacteria, and larger particulate matter from the water being treated. Reverse osmosis can remove many types of dissolved and suspended species from water, including bacteria. The process uses pressure to force the water through the membrane, allowing the water molecules to pass through.

INTENTIONAL POISONING of CITIZENS: FLUORIDE

Two-thirds of the nation's municipal water is fluoridated. Water fluoridation was a bizarre idea that caught on some years ago. It had to do with the strange idea of using the municipal water system to apply fluoride to human teeth. To this day, the subject is hotly contested. Long before I had my calling to the water faith, I saw a strange movie mention of fluoridation. In 1969, Stanley Kubrick produced *Dr. Strangelove*, as I was headed for the high seas and saltwater showers courtesy of the U.S. Navy.

Our own exciting fluoride discussion opens with a scene from Columbia Pictures' strange tale of commies poisoning our water:

Petty Officer Group Captain Mandrake (Peter Sellers), chats with his comrade Strategic Air Command General Jack D. Ripper (Sterling Hayden).

"Ripper: *Mandrake?*

Mandrake: *Yes, Jack?*

Ripper: *Have you ever seen a Commie drink a glass of water?*

Mandrake: *Well, I can't say I have, Jack.*

Ripper: *Vodka, that's what they drink, isn't it? Never water?*

Mandrake: *Well, I-I believe that's what they drink, Jack, yes.*

Ripper: *On no account will a Commie ever drink water, and not without good reason.*

Mandrake: *Oh, eh, yes. I, uhm, can't quite see what you're getting at, Jack.*

Ripper: *Water, that's what I'm getting at, water. Mandrake, water is the source of all life. Seven-tenths of this Earth's surface is water. Why, do you realize that 70 percent of you is water?*

Mandrake: *Good Lord!*

Ripper: *And as human beings, you and I need fresh, pure water to replenish our precious bodily fluids.*

Mandrake: Yes. (he begins to chuckle nervously)

Ripper: Are you beginning to understand?

Mandrake: Yes. (more laughter)

Ripper: Mandrake. Mandrake, have you never wondered why I drink only distilled water, or rainwater, and only pure-grain alcohol?

Mandrake: Well, it did occur to me, Jack, yes.

Ripper: Have you ever heard of a thing called fluoridation. Fluoridation of water?

Mandrake: Uh? Yes, I-I have heard of that, Jack, yes. Yes.

Ripper: Well, do you know what it is?

Mandrake: No, no I don't know what it is, no.

Ripper: Do you realize that fluoridation is the most monstrously conceived and dangerous Communist plot we have ever had to face?

That levity brings us to the serious matter of fluoridated drinking water. Here is an excerpted explanation of the history and virtue of the intentional addition of a poisonous chemical into our municipal and (the tap portion of) bottled water. The pro-fluoride view is presented by The National Institute of Dental and Craniofacial Research (NIDCR) and it is the federal government's lead agency for scientific research on dental, oral and craniofacial health and disease. NIDCR is one department of the National Institutes of Health (NIH) in the U.S. Department of Health and Human Services:

> In 1909 Dr. McKay (r) persuaded the Colorado State Dental Association to invite Dr. Green Vardiman Black (l), one of the nation's most eminent dental researchers, to attend 1909 convention where McKay's findings were to be presented. The two men began joint research and

discovered other areas of the country where brown staining of teeth occurred.

Fluoride research had its beginnings in 1901, when a young dental school graduate named Frederick McKay left the East Coast to open a dental practice in Colorado Springs, Colorado. When he arrived, McKay was astounded to find scores of Colorado Springs natives with grotesque brown stains on their teeth. So severe could these permanent stains be, in fact, sometimes entire teeth were splotched the color of chocolate candy. McKay searched in vain for information on this bizarre disorder. He found no mention of the brown-stained teeth in any of the dental literature of the day. Local residents blamed the problem on any number of strange factors, such as eating too much pork, consuming inferior milk, and drinking calcium-rich water. Thus, McKay took up the gauntlet and initiated research into the disorder himself. His first epidemiological investigations were scuttled by a lack of interest among most area dentists. But McKay persevered and ultimately interested local practitioners in the problem, which was known as Colorado Brown Stain.

A Fruitful Collaboration

McKay's first big break came in 1909, when renowned dental researcher Dr. G.V. Black agreed to come to Colorado Springs and collaborate with him on the mysterious ailment. Black, who had previously scoffed that it was impossible such a disorder could go unreported in the dental literature, was lured West shortly after the Colorado Springs Dental Society conducted a study showing that almost 90 percent of the city's locally born children had signs of the brown stains. When Black arrived in the city, he too was shocked by the prevalence of Colorado Brown Stain in the mouths of native-born residents. He would write later:

'I spent considerable time walking on the streets, noticing the children in their play, attracting their attention and talking with them about their games, etc., for the purpose of studying the general effect of the deformity. I found it prominent in every group of children. One does not have to search for it, for it is continually forcing itself on the attention of the stranger by its persistent prominence. This is much more than a deformity of childhood. If it were only that, it would be of less consequence, but it is a deformity for life.'

Black investigated fluorosis for six years, until his death in 1915. During that period, he and McKay made two crucial discoveries. First, they showed that mottled enamel (as Black referred to the condition) resulted from developmental imperfections in children's teeth. This finding meant that city residents whose permanent teeth had calcified without developing the stains did not risk having their teeth turn brown; young children waiting for their secondary set of teeth to erupt, however, were at high risk. Second, they found that teeth afflicted by Colorado Brown Stain were surprisingly and inexplicably resistant to decay. The two researchers were still a long way from determining the cause of Colorado Brown Stain, but McKay had a theory tucked away in the back of his head. Maybe there was, as some local residents suggested, an ingredient in the water supply that mottled the teeth? Black was skeptical; McKay, though, was intrigued by this theory's prospects.....

McKay collected the samples. And, within months, he had the answer and denouement to his 30-year quest: high levels of water-borne fluoride indeed caused the discoloration of tooth enamel.

New Questions Emerge

Hence, from the curious findings of Churchill's lab assistant, the mystery of the brown stained teeth was cracked. But one mystery often ripples into many others. And shortly after this discovery, PHS scientists started investigating a slew of new and provocative questions about water-borne fluoride. With these PHS investigations, research on fluoride and its effects on tooth enamel began in earnest. The architect of these first fluoride studies was Dr. H. Trendley Dean, head of the Dental Hygiene Unit at the National Institute of Health (NIH). Dean began investigating the epidemiology of fluorosis in 1931. One of his primary research concerns was determining how high fluoride levels could be in drinking water before fluorosis occurred. To determine this, Dean enlisted the help of Dr. Elias Elvove, a senior chemist at the NIH. Dean gave Elvove the hardscrabble task of developing a more accurate method to measure fluoride levels in drinking water. Elvove labored long and hard in his laboratory, and within two years he reported back to Dean with success. He had developed a state-of-the-art method to measure fluoride levels in water with an accuracy of 0.1 parts per million (ppm). With this new method in tow, Dean and his staff set out across the country to compare fluoride levels in drinking water. By the late 1930s, he and his staff had made a critical discovery. Namely, fluoride levels of up to 1.0 ppm in drinking water did not cause enamel fluorosis in most people and only mild enamel fluorosis in a small percentage of people.

Proof That Fluoride Prevents Cavities

This finding sent Dean's thoughts spiraling in a new direction. He recalled from reading McKay's and Black's studies on fluorosis that mottled tooth enamel is unusually resistant to decay. Dean wondered whether adding fluoride to drinking water at physically and cosmetically safe levels would help fight tooth decay. This hypothesis, Dean told his colleagues, would need to be tested. In 1944, Dean got his wish. That year, the City Commission of Grand Rapids, Michigan - after numerous discussions with researchers from the PHS, the Michigan Department of Health, and other public health organizations - voted to add fluoride to its public water supply the following year. In 1945, Grand Rapids became the first city in the world to fluoridate its drinking water. The Grand Rapids water fluoridation study was originally sponsored by the U.S. Surgeon General, but was taken over by the NIDR shortly after the Institute's inception in 1948. During the 15-year project, researchers monitored the rate of tooth decay among Grand Rapids' almost 30,000 schoolchildren. After just 11 years, Dean- who was now director of the NIDR-announced an amazing finding. The caries rate among Grand Rapids children born after fluoride was added to the water supply dropped more than 60 percent. This finding, considering the thousands of participants in the study, amounted to a giant scientific breakthrough that promised to revolutionize dental care, making tooth decay for the first time in history a preventable disease for most people.

A Lasting Achievement

Almost 30 years after the conclusion of the Grand Rapids fluoridation study, fluoride continues to be dental science's main weapon in the battle against tooth decay. Today, just about every toothpaste on the market contains fluoride as its active ingredient; water fluoridation projects currently benefit over 200 million Americans, and 13 million schoolchildren now participate in school-based fluoride mouth rinse programs. As the figures indicate, McKay, Dean, and the others helped to transform dentistry into a prevention-oriented profession. Their drive, in the face of overwhelming adversity, is no less than a remarkable feat of science-an achievement ranking with the other great preventive health measures of our century... (http://www.nidcr.nih.gov/oralhealth/Topics/Fluoride/ TheStoryofFluoridation.htm)

That glorious explanation from a prestigious organization pretty much leaves no room for argument as to the positive aspects of having our water fluoridated, and assists my memories of being forced, at ruler point, to chew a nasty pink fluoride pill in Harvey (Louisiana) Elementary School, with assurances that this was to guarantee my continuing dental health.

There is, alas, another version of the fluoridation story. Fluoride is clearly not a required nutrient, but it has a government recommended AI, or adequate intake, so what the heck is it? To further clarify the toxicity, here we are told what to do in case of an overdose:

> Fluoride is a chemical commonly used to prevent tooth decay. Fluoride overdose occurs when someone takes more than the normal or recommended amount of this substance. This can be by accident or on purpose.
>
> This is for information only and not for use in the treatment or management of an actual overdose. DO NOT use it to treat or manage an actual overdose. If you or someone you are with overdoses, call your local emergency number (such as 911), or your local poison center can be reached directly by calling the national toll-free Poison Help hotline (1-800-222-1222) from anywhere in the United States.
>
> *Poisonous Ingredient*
>
> Fluoride can be harmful in large amounts.
>
> *Where Found*
>
> Fluoride is found in many over-the-counter and prescription products, including:
>
> Certain mouthwashes and toothpastes
>
> Certain vitamins (Tri-Vi-Flor, Poly-Vi-Flor, Vi-Daylin F)
>
> Water that has fluoride added to it
>
> Sodium fluoride liquid and tablets

Fluoride may also be found in other household items, including

Etching cream (also called acid cream, used to etch designs in drinking glasses)

Roach powders

Other products may also contain fluoride.

Symptoms

Symptoms of a fluoride overdose include:

Abdominal pain

Abnormal taste in the mouth (salty or soapy taste)

Convulsions

Diarrhea

Drooling

Eye irritation (if placed in eye)

Headache

Heart attack

Irregular or slow heartbeat

Nausea and vomiting

Shallow breathing

Tremors

Weakness

Before Calling Emergency

Have this information ready:

Person's age, weight, and condition (for example, is the person awake or alert?)

Name of the product (ingredients and strength, if known)

Time it was swallowed

Amount swallowed

Call for help even if you don't know this information.

Poison Control

Your local poison center can be reached directly by calling the national toll-free Poison Help hotline (1-800-222-1222) from anywhere in the United States...

What to Expect at the Emergency Room

Take the container to the hospital with you, if possible.

The health care provider will measure and monitor the person's vital signs, including temperature, pulse, breathing rate, and blood pressure. Symptoms will be treated. The person may receive:

Blood and urine tests

Breathing support, including a tube through the mouth into the lungs, and a breathing machine (ventilator)

Calcium or milk

Chest x-ray

EKG (electrocardiogram, or heart tracing)

Fluids through a vein (by IV)

Laxatives

Medicines to treat symptoms

Tube through the mouth into the stomach to wash out the stomach (gastric lavage)

The above tests and treatments are more likely to be done if someone overdoses on fluoride from household products. They are less likely to be done for an overdose of fluoride from toothpaste and other health products.

Outlook (Prognosis)

How well someone does depend on how much fluoride they swallowed and how quickly they receive treatment. The faster a person gets medical help, the better the chance for recovery.

The amount of fluoride in toothpaste is usually not swallowed in large enough amounts to cause harm.

(http://healthmedicinet.com/ency/article/002650.htm)

The war of intentional water fluoridation of municipal water supplies rages on, and is fought on the ethical, moral political, economic, and safety battle fronts. The opposition argues for the banning of additional fluoridation because there are serious health concerns and the dosage to each individual can never be controlled. This also serves as a compromise of individual rights, as there are no provisions for opting out. The battle started in the '40s and the conspiratorial among us as in our movie *Dr. Strangelove*, cited here, picked up the chase in the '50s and '60s. It continues today on all fronts.

Let's return to the safety and comfort of our movie…

Mandrake patronizes Jack with talk of his own water-drinking habits and personal virility:

> *"Mandrake: Do I look all rancid and clotted? You look at me, Jack. Eh? Look, eh? And I drink a lot of water, you know. I'm what you might call a water man, Jack — that's what I am. And I can swear to you, my boy, swear to you, that there's nothing wrong with my bodily fluids. Not a thing, Jackie."*

WATERFICTION: A sink- top filter will remove chlorine and fluoride form my water.

WATERFACT: The best type of filter to remove chlorine and its byproducts is a combination carbon/KDF adsorption filter (not to be confused with absorption). "Absorption and adsorption are two natural occurring processes that are similar, but not the same: absorption occurs when one material's physical state is absorbed into another materials physical state, while adsorption occurs when one material physically sticks to another material without changing its physical state." (hengyeinc.com)

Pitcher or faucet-mounted water filters do not change fluoride content; reverse osmosis systems can remove 65–95% of fluoride, while distillation removes all fluoride. Some bottled waters contain undeclared fluoride, which can be present naturally in source waters, or if water is sourced from a public supply which has been fluoridated. The FDA states that "bottled water products labeled as de-ionized, purified, demineralized, or distilled have been treated in such a way that they contain no or only trace amounts of fluoride, unless they specifically list fluoride as an added ingredient…"

Now we have beaten the drum of us being intentionally poisoned by our government and trusted municipalities. Now we will paddle on down the stream to enjoy the pavilions of water standards dictated by the aforementioned regulatory bodies and (more trusted) home testing and filtering.

Chapter

8

WATER STANDARDS, HOME TESTING, AND FILTERING

We will explore the depths of drinking water standards, how we can test our water for the myriad of toxins, and how to filter them out. Water toxicity, discussed here at length, ultimately gives way to water scarcity, which, despite the media sensation and conspiracy theories gone wild, is not likely to darken our door in the U.S.A.

Water crises of weather, like Katrina, and the horrors of leaded water, like Flint, are rare in the U.S. Algae crisis is caused by phosphorous runoff. There is no intention here to minimize their reality. One can, however, Google "water crisis in the US" and select "past week" and come up with a host of amazing crises you never dreamed of. Sewage overflow will likely have temporarily paralyzed some areas and will probably continue.

Let's focus, instead, on identifying what is in that water we drink every day and how we can minimize the potential harm living there.

As for water scarcity, broached here on occasion out of necessity, this book strives to be about water cleanliness. About the time the idea of a drought actually catches on, the floods of El Nino fill the aquifers. Presto ... no drought! The avocados and water hungry almond crops are safe, thank God. CNN even stops talking about some water plight here in the U.S. as the aquifers are full and forgotten for a time. Water rights activists put away their signs for another day, and get right with the party. Amazing that a good old rainstorm can transform a protest.

The point is that it is hard to stay concerned about our personal drinking water for very long, and even harder to commit time to study and dollars to get it right. It drops from our consciousness.

Globally there are certainly areas of catastrophic drinking water scarcity, and climate and politics are the culprits. I witnessed this first hand in many instances. In most cases of scarcity, there is still not a problem of lack of water, but one of distribution. Because of its 8 pounds per gallon, incompressibility, and absolute necessity, we have to remain aware of our good water fortunes here in our beloved U.S.A. and count our blessings. Our objective is to make it all better.

We have to commit a bit of time to understand, and money to get our own personal "water plant" in place and then enjoy it. It is quite empowering to take our water purity into our own hands and understand that the government is ineffective in their alleged job of water cleanliness. Fluoride is added intentionally! Lead from water mains and in much of our personal plumbing, in the guise of solder on our copper pipes, demands our personal attention!

According to one 2002 survey of 1,000 households, an estimated 56% of us Americans drank water straight from the tap and an additional 37% drank tap water after filtering it. 74% of Americans said they bought bottled water. (I feel certain that the remaining 26% buy water in bottles, maybe in secret, at night.) After all, our consumption of bottled water, discussed at length earlier, defines in part who we are as human beings. 86% of us rely on our trusted Sewage and Water Board to get water as far as the meter, the remaining 14% are "self supplied," presumably from wells. (http://water. usgs.gov/edu/wups.html)

Every sip from any source takes us into the gaudy casino of water purity roulette!

The cylinder is spun at the water meter, and the gun is pointed at us. The government has exhaustively regulated and not necessarily fixed the water at that point of demarcation:

Drinking Water Standards

To review: The Environmental Protection Agency (EPA) identifies contaminants to regulate in drinking water. The Agency sets regulatory limits for the amounts of certain contaminants in water provided by public water systems. These standards apply to their side of the meter!

Primary Contaminants

The National Primary Drinking Water Regulations (NPDWRs or primary standards) are legally enforceable standards that apply to public water systems. Primary standards protect public health by limiting the levels of contaminants in drinking water. Visit the site below of regulated contaminants for details.

- Microorganisms
- Disinfectants
- Disinfection Byproducts
- Inorganic Chemicals
- Organic Chemicals
- Radionuclides

Secondary Contaminants

> EPA established National Secondary Drinking Water Regulations that set non-mandatory water quality standards for 15 contaminants. EPA does not enforce these "secondary maximum contaminant levels (SCML)." They are established only as guidelines to assist public water systems in managing their drinking water for aesthetic considerations, such as taste, color, and odor. These contaminants are not considered to present a risk to human health at the SCML. For exhaustive details: https://www.epa.gov/dwstandardsregulations

Why set secondary standards?

These contaminants are not health threatening at the public water systems only need to test for them on a voluntary basis. Then why it is necessary to set secondary standards?

EPA believes that if these contaminants are present in your water at levels above these standards, the contaminants may cause the water to appear cloudy or colored, or to taste or smell bad. This may cause a great number of people to stop using water from their public water system even though the water is actually safe to drink.

Secondary standards are set to give public water systems some guidance on removing these chemicals to levels that are below what most people will find to be noticeable.

What problems are caused by these contaminants?

There are a wide variety of problems related to secondary contaminants.

These problems can be grouped into three categories:

- Aesthetic effects — undesirable tastes or odors;
- Cosmetic effects — effects which do not damage the body but are still undesirable
- Technical effects — damage to water equipment or reduced effectiveness of treatment for other contaminants. These effects are shown in the table below.

Aesthetic Effects

Odor and taste are useful indicators of water quality even though odor-free water is not necessarily safe to drink. Odor is also an indicator of the effectiveness of different kinds of treatment. However, present methods of measuring taste and odor are still fairly subjective and the task of identifying an unacceptable level for each chemical in different waters requires more study. Also, some contaminant odors are noticeable even when present in extremely small amounts. It is usually very expensive and often impossible to identify, much less remove, the odor-producing substance.

- Standards related to odor and taste: Chloride, Copper, Foaming Agents, Iron, Manganese pH, Sulfate, Threshold Odor Number (), Total Dissolved Solids, Zinc

Color may be indicative of dissolved organic material, inadequate treatment, high disinfectant demand, and the potential for the production of excess amounts of disinfectant by-products. Inorganic contaminants such as metals are also common causes of color. In general, the point of consumer complaint is variable over a range from five to 30 color units. Most people find color objectionable over 15 color units. Rapid changes in color levels may provoke more citizen complaints than a relatively high, constant color level.

- Standards related to color: Aluminum, Color, Copper, Iron, Manganese, Total Dissolved Solids.

Foaming is usually caused by detergents and similar substances when water has been agitated or aerated as in many faucets. An off-taste described as oily, fishy, or perfume-like is commonly associated with foaming. However, these tastes and odors may be due to the breakdown of waste products rather than the detergents themselves.

- Standards related to foaming: Foaming Agents

Cosmetic effects

Skin discoloration is a cosmetic effect related to silver ingestion. This effect, called argyria, does not impair body function. It has never been found to be caused by drinking water in the United States. A standard has been set, however, because silver is used as an antibacterial agent in many home water treatment devices and so presents a potential problem which deserves attention.

•   Standard related to this effect: Silver

Tooth discoloration and/or pitting is caused by excess fluoride exposures during the formative period prior to eruption of the teeth in children. The secondary standard of 2.0 is intended as a guideline for an upper boundary level in areas which have high levels of naturally occurring fluoride. The level of the S was set based upon a balancing of the beneficial effects of protection from tooth decay and the undesirable effects of excessive exposures leading to discoloration. Information about the Centers for Disease Control's (CDC) recommendations regarding optimal fluoridation levels and the beneficial effects for protection from tooth decay can be found on CDC's site: http://www.cdc.gov/fluoridation/

•   Standard related to this effect: Fluoride

Technical effects

Corrosivity, and staining related to corrosion, not only affect the aesthetic quality of water, but may also have significant economic implications. Other effects of corrosive water, such as the corrosion of iron and copper, may stain household fixtures and impart objectionable metallic taste and red or blue-green color to the water supply. Corrosion of distribution system pipes can reduce water flow.

- Standards related to corrosion and staining: Chloride, Copper, Corrosivity, Iron, Manganese, pH, Total Dissolved Solids, Zinc

Scaling and sedimentation are other processes which have economic impacts. Scale is a mineral deposit which builds up on the insides of hot water pipes, boilers, and heat exchangers, restricting or even blocking water flow. Sediments are loose deposits in the distribution system or home plumbing.

- Standards related to scale and sediments: Iron, pH, Total Dissolved Solids, Aluminum

(https://www.epa.gov/dwstandardsregulations/secondary-drinking-water-standards-guidance-nuisance-chemicals)

Conspicuously absent from the list above is mention of pharmaceutical contaminants from the annual 4.3 billion prescribed medications that wind up in our drinking water.

Chemical and Engineering News reports that using recycled city water for our vegetable gardens and agricultural needs, boosts traceable quantities of carbamazine, an anti-epileptic drug commonly detected in wastewater. That drug is being found in the water as a result of drain disposal of unused medications.

(http://cen.acs.org/articles/94/web/2016/04/Vegetables-grown-treated-wastewater-boost.html)

Despite vague assurances of purity, and primary and secondary regulations, we are left at our meter with promises. Now we have to get serious and purify our water at the tap and bottle because, while busy establishing all of those tedious regulations, perhaps our government allowed something bad to slip in!

So who you gonna call? Now we are all indoctrinated into the club of taking responsibility for our own water. We are committed to correct our water at point-of-use! Now we will learn how to proceed to minimize the risk of unclean water getting into us. With our new-found knowledge of what toxins that tap, bottle, or fountain may dispense, we will study water purification methods we can use to assure that we are drinking safe water.

We are confronted with choices of under-sink filtration, refrigerator filters, shower, faucet, and pitcher filters. Terms like single stage, multi stage, and simplex designs further obscure our mission.

We may have already bought a carload of filters and put them on the faucets and maybe in the showers, or perhaps we are just starting down that road. Either way we are now all soldiers in the war for pure personal drinking water. Our first mission in the process is to test the water.

WATER TESTING

Amazon and Home Depot abound with do-it-yourself (DIY) home test kits.

Home Testing:

For around $30.00 we can test for the following, with one kit:

- 10 Minute Lead Test: Lead can cause developmental, neurological, gastrointestinal and reproductive damage.
- Pesticide Test: Pesticides can be linked to increased cancer rates and organ damage.
- Bacteria/Coliform Test: Certain strains of bacteria can cause serious illness or death.
- Iron: High levels of iron can destroy your property and create a bad taste.
- Nitrates: Nitrates can cause developmental issues.
- Nitrites: Nitrites can cause developmental issues.
- Chlorine Level: Chlorine can increase your risk of cancer.
- Copper: High levels of copper can cause gastrointestinal issues and has been associated with liver damage and kidney disease.
- Alkalinity: High levels of alkaline can cause gastrointestinal issues.
- pH Test: High pH levels can cause plumbing and property damage.

- Water Hardness: Water hardness can create a bad taste and cause property damage.

Lab testing is more thorough and there are water testing services that send you a reminder, a sterile sample bottle, and a bill at some interval.

Now that testing is complete we can proceed to understand the various methods of filtration, and their respective limitations. This will brace us in advance for the onslaught of filtration choices that we will be confronted with as we advance our water purity project.

FILTRATION PHYSICS

What is a micron? Medical Definition of micron.: a unit of length equal to one millionth of a meter—called also micrometer, mu.

(http://www.merriam-webster.com/dictionary/micron)

Water filters are "Micron Rated." This is simply the size of the spaces between pieces of the filter material. The idea is that a 10 micron filter will allow more contaminants to pass through than a 5 micron filter, and, consequently, cost more. The flow-through rate of water is also reduced in direct proportion to the smaller micron rating of the filter.

Viruses: 0.005 to 0.1 microns

Bacteria: 0.1 to 10 microns

Protozoa and cysts: 1 to 20 microns

But Wait.. the filter industry often omits the distinction ABSOLUTE vs NOMINAL in describing their filters. Absolute means that the filter will remove absolutely all particles down to the rated size, whereas nominal means removal of down to that size!

It is important that any filter company you choose is specifically certified by NSF of WQA. The NSF mark:

assures consumers, retailers and regulators that products have been rigorously tested to comply with all standard requirements.

The NSF certification mark on a product means that the product complies with all standard requirements. NSF conducts periodic unannounced inspections and product testing to verify that the product continues to comply with the standard.

The mark also provides:

- Knowledge that an impartial review against established criteria or guidelines has been conducted
- Evidence that product labeling and claims have been objectively reviewed by a trusted third party
- A way to differentiate your product from your competitors' and gain advantage in the market
- Evidence of your organization's company-wide commitment to quality, compliance and safety
- Backing by a team of professionals dedicated to public health and safety operating in more than 150 countries around the world… (nsf.org)

WQA: "The Water Quality Association (WQA) is a not-for-profit international trade association representing the residential, commercial and industrial water treatment industry. WQA maintains a close dialogue with other organizations representing different aspects of the water industry in order to best serve consumers, government officials, and industry members. WQA is a resource and information source, a voice for the industry, an educator for professionals, a laboratory for product testing, and a communicator to the public." (http://www.wqa.org)

WATER FILTRATION TYPES:

Carbon/Activated Carbon/Carbon Block:

"Activated carbon works via a process called adsorption, whereby pollutant molecules in the fluid to be treated are trapped inside the pore structure of the carbon substrate. Carbon filtering is commonly used for water purification.

"Active charcoal carbon filters are most effective at removing chlorine, sediment, volatile organic compounds (VOCs), taste and odor from water. They are not effective at removing minerals, salts, and dissolved inorganic compounds...Typical particle sizes that can be removed by carbon filters range from 0.5 to 50 micrometers. The particle size will be used as part of the filter description. The efficacy of a carbon filter is also based upon the flow rate regulation. When the water is allowed to flow through the filter at a slower rate, the contaminants are exposed to the filter media for a longer amount of time.

"There are 2 predominant types of carbon filters used in the filtration industry: powdered block filters and granular activated filters. In general, carbon block filters are more effective at removing a larger number of contaminants, based upon the increased surface area of carbon. Many carbon filters also use secondary media such as silver to prevent bacteria growth within the filter. Alternatively, the activated carbon itself may be impregnated with silver to provide this bacteriostatic property..." (https://en.wikipedia.org/wiki/Carbon_filtering)

Ceramic filters: are an inexpensive and effective type of water filter, that rely on the small pore size of ceramic material to filter dirt, debris, and bacteria out of water. They do not remove toxic chemicals, they can remove sediments and cysts. (https://en.wikipedia.org/wiki/Ceramic_water_filter)

Deionization filters: The process used for removal of all dissolved salts from water is referred to as deionization. Deionization requires the flow of water through two ion exchange materials in order to affect the removal of all salt content.

They do not remove microorganisms, trihlomethanes, or other VOCs. (http://www.tdsmeter.com/what-is?id=0015)

Fibredyne block: Fibredyne block filters are a common water filtration technology. It is a proprietary type of carbon block filter. It is said to have a higher sediment holding capacity than other carbon block filters.

(https://www.sharecare.com/health/water-liquid-nutrient/what-is-fibredyne-block-filter)

Microfiltration/Ultrafiltration: Membranes with a pore size of 0.1 – 10 μm perform microfiltration. Microfiltration membranes remove all bacteria. Only part of the viral contamination is caught up in the process, even though viruses are smaller than the pores of a micro filtration membrane. This is because viruses can attach themselves to bacterial biofilm.

Micro filtration can be implemented in many different water treatment processes when particles with a diameter greater than 0.1 mm need to be removed from a liquid.

For complete removal of viruses, ultra-filtration is required. The pores of ultra-filtration membranes can remove particles of 0.001 – 0.1 μm from fluids.

(http://www.lenntech.com/microfiltration-and-ultrafiltration.htm)

Mechanical Filters: Like ceramic filters, these filters have small holes that remove cysts and sediments, but do not work to remove chemical contaminants. Mechanical filtration systems include cartridge sediment filters, media and multimedia filters, and precoat filters.

Our expertise in what different filters do for us leads us to Alternative Water Purification. Methods like distillation and reverse osmosis are effective for removal of chloride, fluoride, viruses, bacteria, total dissolved solids, and other inorganic substances.

Alternative Water Purification Methods:

Boiling: By boiling drinking water, you lose some of the water, the process of which further concentrates chemicals or harmful solids already there. The good news for boiling is that parasites and bacteria may be killed in the process. "For E. coli bring water to a rolling boil for one minute (at elevations above 6.500 feet, boil for 3 minutes) Water should then be allowed to cool, stored in a clean sanitized container with a tight cover, and refrigerated." (www.cdc.gov/healthywater/drinking/private/wells/disease/e_coli.html)

Distillation: Heats water to vapor and condenses the steam back into water. Removes chemicals that have a higher boiling point than water, and when used with a charcoal filter, removes many bacteria, fluoride, chlorine, and volatile organic chemicals. VOCs. Effectiveness varies between manufacturers based on addition of filtration configurations and venting.

Ion Exchange: Resins are used to remove poisonous (e.g. copper) and heavy metal (e.g. lead or cadmium) ions from solution, replacing them with more innocuous ions, such as sodium and potassium. Few ion-exchange resins remove chlorine or organic contaminants from water – this is usually done by using an activated charcoal filter mixed in with the resin. There are some ion-exchange resins that do remove organic ions, such as MIEX (magnetic ion-exchange) resins. Domestic water purification resin is not usually recharged – the resin is discarded when it can no longer be used. Resins [remove contaminants] by using an activated charcoal filter mixed in with the resin. (https://en.wikipedia.org/wiki/Ion-exchange_resin#Water_purification)

Ozone: Ozone (Ozonation) kills bacteria and other microorganisms and is often used in conjunction with other filtering technologies. It is not effective in removing chemical contaminants. Ozone will not remove nitrates (typical when water is contaminated by fertilizer run off), sodium, sulfates, total dissolved solids, chlorides, and fluoride. These contaminants can be removed by reverse osmosis or distillation.

Reverse Osmosis (RO): RO systems use many times the water they produce. It is a "water purification technology that uses a semipermeable membrane to remove ions, molecules, and larger particles from drinking water. In reverse osmosis, an applied pressure is used to overcome osmotic pressure, a colligative property, that is driven by chemical potential differences of the solvent, athermodynamic parameter. Reverse osmosis can remove many types of dissolved and suspended species from water, including bacteria, and is used...in the production of potable water. The result is that the solute is retained on the pressurized side of the membrane and the pure solvent is allowed to pass to the other side. To be "selective", this membrane should not allow large molecules or ions through the pores (holes), but should allow smaller components of the solution (such as solvent molecules) to pass freely. (https://en.wikipedia.org/wiki/Reverse_osmosis)

UV (ultraviolet): Ultraviolet germicidal irradiation (UVGI) is a disinfection method that uses short-wavelength ultraviolet (UV-C) light to kill or inactivate microorganisms by destroying nucleic acids and disrupting their DNA, leaving them unable to perform vital cellular functions.[1] UVGI is used in.. water purification. (https://en.wikipedia.org/wiki/Ultraviolet_germicidal_irradiation)

Water Softeners: Water softening is the removal of calcium, magnesium, and certain other metal cations in hard water. The resulting soft water is more compatible with soap and extends the lifetime of plumbing. Water softening is usually achieved using lime softening or ion-exchange resins. (https://en.wikipedia.org/wiki/Water_softening)

NSF provides to us consumers their "guide to contaminant reduction guide claims." Their ambiguous title is better translated as: what may be in our water and what methods they recommend to remove it.

"All sources of drinking water can contain some contaminants. At low levels, most of these contaminants are not considered to be harmful by agencies such as the U.S. Environmental Protection Agency (EPA), Health Canada or World Health Organization. Some contaminants are naturally occurring in the environment, including radon, radium and arsenic. People, animals and industry can also add contaminants to our water supplies."

For a list of contaminants, check out the full interactive NSF site: *http://www.nsf.org/consumer-resources/what-is-nsf-certification/water-filters-treatment-certification/contaminant-reduction-claims-guide*

Now we have identified what exact contaminants the government is monitoring, and our obligation to assume full responsibility for our water purity at the meter inbound. We reviewed exactly

- what to test for in our drinking water
- filtration systems and exactly what they remove
- alternative systems we can buy to purify our personal water supply.
- interactive site by contaminant from nsf.org

WATERFICTION: Distilling water removes essential minerals that our bodies need.

WATERFACT: "This assertion is made because distilled water doesn't have any minerals of its own. However, most of the minerals we take in come from food, not water. And the fact is that your kidneys do a fine job of keeping your minerals in proper balance. As long as your kidneys are functioning normally, you'll have no problems drinking distilled water." (drdavidwilliams.com)

What if there was a way to actually rise above the infrastructure and all of its inherent contaminants entirely? Visors down, get ready for the carrier launch into the world of Water Machines.

Chapter

9

WATER MACHINES

We have clearly identified the water infrastructure as the repository of the many toxic offenders attacking our fragile personal drinking water. Some of these toxic chemicals are intentionally added to our water (as in the case of fluoride, chlorine, and ammonia)!

We have discussed methods of removing the toxins at strategic points prior to our ingestion of the water. As we looked deeper into the pool darkly we discovered that, despite our best filtering efforts, toxins could well be present in their elusive and progressively microscopic quantities.

Good news! We also have the option to install a water machine that will extract moisture from the air, and *under conditions of adequate relative humidity*, distribute it to us, having never picked up any toxic chemicals, pollutants, or radiation.

These machines, called atmospheric water generators (AWG), come at a cost, but they certainly avoid the infrastructure entirely and the pollutants residing in the highly regulated and sporadically purified municipal water systems.

These machines, hardly magical or new, extract water from the air. We can refer to this process as *changing the phase* of water from gas (in the air) to a liquid.

Various configurations of these "water generators" actually micro-filter the air at the intake, remove the airborne pollutants, then extract the water. Several methods are then employed to further purify the now extracted, stored water.

The AWG concept also enjoyed some fame in the movies:

> In the *Dune* series, Fremen on the desert world Arrakis collected water from the atmosphere on a massive scale by erecting wind traps that funneled dew-laden air into cool underground caverns.
>
> In *Star Wars*, Luke Skywalker's family on Tatooine used atmospheric water generation on their moisture farm.
>
> In the *Star Trek: The Next Generation* episode 'The Inner Light', Captain Picard suggests building 'atmospheric condensers' for a planet experiencing prolonged drought.
>
> (https://en.wikipedia.org/wiki/ Atmospheric_water_generator#In_fiction)

These future era movie depictions of the concept overlook the realities of AWGs in our own moments in time.

For our atmospheric water generation history briefing, the Incas were able to sustain their culture above the rain line by collecting dew and channeling it to cisterns for later distribution. Historical records indicate the use of water-collecting fog fences. Cloth was hung outside to collect dew in the ancient world.

How do the modern era AWGs work?

Air is passed over a cooled coil, causing air to condense causing moisture. The extracted moisture and water is collected and purified by various methods, i.e. ozonation, UV, filtration. The rate of water production depends on the altitude, ambient temperature, humidity, the volume of air passing over the coil, and the machine's capacity to cool the coil, thus condensing the air. These systems reduce air temperature, which in turn reduces the air's capacity to carry water vapor and forces the moisture into water and is collected.

Atmospheric Water Generators become more effective as relative humidity and air temperature increase. As a rule of thumb, cooling condensation atmospheric water generators do not work efficiently when the temperature falls below 18.3°C (65°F) or the relative humidity drops below 30%. This means they are relatively inefficient when located inside air-conditioned offices or any confined spaces as eventually most of the moisture in that space will be removed. The cost-effectiveness of an AWG depends on the capacity of the machine, local humidity and temperature conditions and the cost to power the unit.

New emerging technology utilize the Peltier effect of semi-conducting materials in which one side of the semi-conducting material heats while the other side cools. In this application, air is forced over the cooling fins on the side that cools which lowers the temperature of the air to its dew point, causing water to condense. The resulting water is then collected. Due to the solid-state nature of the semi-conducting material and the lower power usage, some of these new designs use solar energy panels as the power source.

The drinking water generation capacity of some AWMs can be enhanced in low humidity ambient air conditions, first by using the evaporative cooler with a brackish water supply to increase the air humidity near to dew point condition. Thus drinking water is generated using brackish water without depending entirely on ambient air humidity by the water generator..."

(https://en.wikipedia.org/wiki/Atmospheric_water_generator)

AWGs will make water in lower humidity environments, but that is in exchange for more watts! The formula is best expressed as "watts = gallons." There is no free ride!

Atmospheric water generators (AWGs) have been with us since the days of the first air conditioners, although they went unrecognized. That water gurgling out of our massive window units, long before the advent of central air, was actually water! For many modern versions of the machines, many suppliers make dubious claims of having *invented* the technology, when in actuality they are cousins of window air conditioners, dehumidifiers, and central air units. The enemies of this air condensing operation are low temperatures, low humidity, and cost of electricity. Low humidity areas are usually places starving for water, i.e., outback Australia, Africa, the Middle East, etc. There is a company that has developed the solution by increasing the humidity in the air prior to cooling and thus condensing. This operation is discussed later in the book.

To better understand AWGs, we have to go back to general science class for a briefing on the water that lives in our air. At any moment, the atmosphere contains an astounding ".37.5 *million billion* gallons of water, in the invisible vapor phase. This is enough water to cover the entire surface of the Earth (land and ocean) with one inch of rain. What's more, this amount of water is recycled 40 times each year in what is known as the hydrological cycle, explained earlier. That means a water vapor molecule has an average residence time in the atmosphere of only nine days: the raindrop that fell on your head last Tuesday on average had evaporated into the atmosphere nine days before..." (http://whyfiles.org/2010/how-much-water-is-in-the-atmosphere/)

The early days of AWGs often included the sarcastic adage "trade a gallon of fuel oil for a gallon of water...." Over time that has changed, but, although an exaggeration, our desperation for clean water brings this into practicality.

The reality of AWG technology is that conditions of water vapor density, dew point, relative humidity, temperature, cost of watts, and variations of water demand are constantly in flux. Quantifying the cost per gallon of water generated by this method is dependent on widely changing values.

Where are water-from-air systems practical? "Water -from- Air machines (AWGs) produce water year-round in locations near sea level between latitudes 30° N and 30° S…" (*Water-From-Air Quick Guide: Second Edition* by Roland V. Wahlgren, published in June 1996.)

Innovative power generation methodologies highlight the increasing practicality of AWGs. Living with the energy cost in exchange for fairly pristine water is sounding like a better idea for many. In the world of alternative, renewable energy generation, there are amazing developments in wind, solar, biomass, geo-thermal, and hydro-electric energy sources. These technologies are readily applicable to the world of atmospheric water production but the inescapable formula remains: Watts = Litres.

The likely world leader in this technology is an Australian company, World Environmental Solutions Pty Ltd, who pioneered during what in Australia was labelled the *Millennium Drought*: a 10-year affair in Australia in the early to mid 2000s. The result was a company that realized making water was desired as drinking water in many cases but the normal method was cost-prohibitive, with electricity costs soaring. One thing was a certain obstacle: the "Watts = Liters" formula. This company today is furthering research and development into its systems of water from the air using minimal power/electricity.

Their water booster (WB) can double the RH at sites where normal operation of an AWG would be inefficient and not advised. That is, the WB can alter 20% RH into 43% RH prior to condensing or 40% RH into 83% RH prior to condensing. (Patent applied for.) This is a real issue for the Sub-Sahara, outback Australia and other arid areas.

The company also has patented its HydroGel filter system, which uses hydrogels impregnated into the filter material, to absorb moisture as air passed through it; as a small amount of electrical power was periodically applied to the filter sub-straight to "desorb" the moisture from the hydro gels. This pulsing effect resulted in water from the air with minimal energy usage.

The company's mainstream development was by use of an air cooled system known as a **MultiGen.** This consisted of a multi-patented air cooled absorption chiller and an air cooled AWM operated free from the waste heat of a Turbine or reciprocating generator exhaust. The byproduct of this process is to provide cool, air-conditioned air to a space, while making water, all operated from waste energy of an existing Generator, to activate the process they use to operate the condensing cycle. This process dramatically drops the use of electricity by some 95%, as the energy source is waste heat captured.

This particular company has a patented system using Hydrogel filters. These hydrogels have the ability to absorb moisture as the air passes through the filter impregnated with Hydrogel substance. Upon a small electrical charge the hydrogel "desorbs" the moisture. This pulsing system can be used in front of most AC systems air intake and thus produce water for a very low cost and at very low RH normally necessary for AWG operation. While still in the R&D phase, prototypes are in operation as proof of concept.

But wait! A latter day solution revisits the bygone era of fog fences, mentioned above. This method is completely passive, requiring no external energy source other than naturally occurring temperature variations.

Modern era fog fence efforts include MIT's recent project to commercialize atmospheric water harvest:

> In some of this planet's driest regions, where rainfall is rare or even nonexistent, a few specialized plants and insects have devised ingenious strategies to provide themselves with the water necessary for life: They pull it right out of the air, from fog that drifts in from warm oceans nearby.
>
> Now researchers at MIT, working in collaboration with colleagues in Chile, are seeking to mimic that trick on a much larger scale, potentially supplying significant quantities of clean, potable water in places where there are few alternatives.
>
> Fog harvesting, essentially atmospheric water generation, is not a new idea: Systems to make use of this airborne potable water already exist now in at least 17 nations. But

the new research shows that their efficiency in a mild fog condition can be improved by at least fivefold, making them far more feasible and practical than existing versions.

The new findings have just been published online by the journal *Langmuir*, a publication of the American Chemical Society, in a paper by MIT postdoc Kyoo-Chul Park PhD '13, MIT alumnus Shreerang Chhatre PhD '13, graduate student Siddarth Srinivasan, chemical engineering professor Robert Cohen, and mechanical engineering professor Gareth McKinley.

Fog-harvesting systems generally consist of a vertical mesh, sort of like an oversized tennis net. Key to efficient harvesting of the tiny airborne droplets of fog are three basic parameters, the researchers found: the size of the filaments in those nets, the size of the holes between those filaments, and the coating applied to the filaments.

Most existing systems turn out to be far from optimal, Park says. Made of woven polyolefin mesh — a kind of plastic that is easily available and inexpensive — they tend to have filaments and holes that are much too large. As a result, they may extract only about 2 percent of the water available in a mild fog condition, whereas the new research shows that a finer mesh could extract 10 percent or more, Park says. Multiple nets deployed one behind another could then extract even more, if so desired.

While some of the organisms that harvest fog do so using solid surfaces — such as the carapace of the Namib beetle, native to the Namib desert of southern Africa — permeable mesh structures are much more effective because the wind-blown fog droplets tend to be deflected around solid surfaces, Park says. Thus, a woven mesh structure resembling a window screen turns out to be most effective. With the right chemical coating, fog droplets that form on the screen then slide down to be collected at the bottom and are funneled into buckets or tanks...

The researchers found that controlling the size and structure of the mesh and the physical and chemical composition of this coating was essential to increasing the fog-collecting efficiency. Detailed calculations and laboratory tests indicate that the best performance comes from a mesh made of stainless-steel filaments about three or four times the thickness of a human hair, and with a spacing of about twice that between fibers. In addition, the mesh is dip-coated, using a solution that decreases a characteristic called contact-angle hysteresis. This allows small droplets to more easily slide down into the collecting gutter as soon as they form, before the wind blows them off the surface and back into the fog stream.

While the systems currently deployed in the coastal mountains at the edge of the Atacama Desert tend to yield a few liters of drinking water per day for each square meter of mesh, the theoretical calculations show that newly designed systems operating in the strong winds and dense fogs that form along the Chilean coast at certain times of the year could yield up to 12 liters per day or more, the researchers say.

In collaboration with researchers at the Pontifical Catholic University in Santiago, Chile, the MIT researchers have recently installed a variety of test screens made of different materials on hilltops in a semi-arid region north of Santiago, an area that sees very little rainfall, but which is regularly enshrouded in a strong windblown coastal fog called *camanchaca* rolling in from the Pacific Ocean. The team is currently carrying out a yearlong test to study the durability and water yield of different configurations.

Maria Tou '14, an MIT undergraduate, worked with the team in Chile, helping to install instrumentation that can observe the fluid mechanics associated with the fog droplets as they collect, grow and coalesce on the meshes.

Large mesh structures, of hundreds of square meters each, could be set up relatively inexpensively; once in place, they cost virtually nothing to operate. They consume no energy, needing only an occasional brushing to remove particles of grit and bugs. "The operating cost is essentially zero," McKinley says, because "nature has already done the hard work of evaporating the water, desalinating it and condensing the droplets. We just have to collect it."

Chilean investigators have estimated that if just 4 percent of the water contained in the fog could be captured, that would be sufficient to meet all of the water needs of that nation's four northernmost regions, encompassing the entire Atacama Desert area. And with the MIT-designed system, Park points out, 10 percent of the fog moisture in the air passing through the new fog collector system can potentially be captured.

Daniel Beysens, director of the Physics and Mechanics of Heterogeneous Media Laboratory at EPSCI in Paris, who was not involved in this research, says, "This is a very important paper for anybody who wants to get water from fog. The authors have performed a thorough theoretical and experimental investigation of the influence on the final water yield of the structure of a fog net. ... Their study is a breakthrough in the design of fog collectors."

The research was supported by a Samsung scholarship, the MIT-Legatum Center for Entrepreneurship and Development, MIT's MISTI-Chile program, and the Xerox Foundation.

(http://news.mit.edu/2013/
how-to-get-fresh-water-out-of-thin-air-0830)

Perhaps the era of getting pristine drinking water from fog is near.

WATERFICTION: Atmospheric Water Generators (AWGs) are the solution to municipal water supply issues of drinking water purity.

WATERFACT: "There are recent technological breakthroughs in the efficiencies of large commercial AWGs. These drastic improvements in versatility and performance make these "next-gen" AWGs the logical choice for modernization of aging infrastructures. These highly engineered and patented machines now offer operation in environments of great variations in atmospheric conditions.

"Constantly changing water demand requires storage solutions, and water in storage demands constant purification solutions, included in the new era machines. Very recent technological advancements in commercialization of municipal AWGs is happening now and requires expert engineering and installation solutions. AWGs are now competitive in the market formerly dominated by filtration based systems." (http://www.atmosphericwaterworks.com)

Now our growing knowledge base includes a way to *completely avoid* the infrastructure and its shortcomings entirely, through the use of AWGs. If MIT has their way, hydrating with fog may also contribute to our personal drinking water future!

Water is happening. It is the *now thing*. Let's invite our broker to accompany us as we enter the world of investing in the myriad of water enterprises.

Chapter

10

WATER INVESTMENT

Water is not officially a commodity, that is: qualified, benchmarked, reported, and traded on exchanges. "Commodities were (are) things of value, of uniform quality, that were produced in large quantities by many different producers ... considered equivalent..." (wikipedia.org/wiki/commodity)

Our newly raised awareness of the many issues with drinking water brings us to the idea that we can contribute to (and profit from) solutions through carefully planned investments in the water space.

Water toxicity makes Olympians deathly ill in Rio, and traffic is rerouted around broken water mains in good old Manhattan. Google "water crisis" and get over 12,900,000 results in 0.47 seconds.

One of the favorite movies of investors is *The Big Short*. The movie, and the book it was based on, focused on the Great Recession, which was triggered by the housing crisis, and the very small group of people who saw it coming very clearly. These people were the ones who made vast fortunes because of their insight. One of those people was Michael Burry. The last line in the movie sums it up, printed on a placard, is "Michael Burry is focusing all of his trading on one commodity: Water."

We have taken our study of the impossibly broad subject of drinking water from inside of us to outside in huge pipes. Pursuant to our aroused interest in water, let's review some of its many complexions covered herein:

Chapter 1   elaborated on the importance of hydrating and the many health risks associated with failing to do so.

Chapter 2   described the inescapable necessity: a complete renovation of our entire water infrastructure. (The necessary funding to accomplish this feat rivals the national defense budget).

Chapter 3   discussed at length the economic vibrancy enjoyed by the bottled water industry.

Chapter 4   addressed the bewildering complexity of toxic chemicals, and the regulatory issues facing local and national governmental agencies in their pursuit of providing clean drinking water through regulation.

Chapter 5   provided inescapable evidence of the fracking process making its negative contribution to our fragile drinking water resources.

Chapter 6   raised the possibility of lead in our own personal water systems, resulting from decaying infrastructure and also from our own plumbing.

Chapter 7   called into question the value of municipalities adding chlorine, fluoride, and other additives into our personal water systems.

Chapter 8   taught us all about various filtration methods.

Chapter 9   explored the possibility of using dollars to buy watts to power machines that make water and avoid the infrastructure entirely.

So, now that we have a good overview and understanding of all of the challenges and difficulties, we ask ourselves the obvious question of what action should we take, if any? With the variety of problems and the growing focus on the issues, there are always those who recognize what is happening and are working on the various solutions.

Remember, this is America, and do not underestimate the resourcefulness of the problem solvers among us. When you believe there is no solution to all of these problems and that we are doomed, always think about the Great Horse Manure Crisis of 1894. What is that? I'm glad you asked.

How many times have you heard that "If this trend continues, the result will be disaster. We are going off the cliff"? The subject can be just about any problem, but the pattern of reaction is the same. People take a current trend and extrapolate it into the future as the basis for their gloomy and doom predictions.

The fundamental problem with most predictions of any kind is that they make a very serious false assumption: that things will go on as they are. People who make these assumptions overlook the very basics of economics and human nature: that, given any problem, people have the insight to see the incentives, and react accordingly. Solutions magically appear.

Now, for the Great Horse Manure Crisis of 1894. At that point in time all of the major cities have the same problem. None worse than London, which was then the largest city in the world, and was still rapidly growing. All of the goods and services were delivered by horse drawn vehicles. All personal transportation in cabs and buses were horse drawn. London had over 100,000 horses in the city on a daily basis, walking and running in the streets of the city, and depositing manure along the way.

In the streets of New York it was estimated that 2.5 million pounds of horse manure was left in the streets every day. Pundits of the day said that urban civilization was doomed. In 1898 the first international urban-planning conference began in New York City. The conference was scheduled to last for ten days. The participants ended the conference after three days, since no one could come up with a solution to the horse problem. They saw that as cities grew, more and more horses would be needed, which meant more stables on valuable land, more land would be needed to grow hay, less land would be available to grow food for people, and not one delegate could think of a solution to the horse manure problem. The *London Times* predicted that, in fifty years, every street in London would be covered in nine feet of horse manure.

The last time I was in London, I did not see any horse manure. What happened? A guy named Henry Ford happened, and all the horse manure went away.

Rest assured that the water problems will be solved. There are lots of Henry Fords working on them; some solutions are obvious and some are not so obvious at the moment.

So if we are not inventors or water solution problem solvers, how can we participate in the birth of the great water phoenix?

We see the following segments in the water industry that have potential for investment:

1. Water Utilities
2. Infrastructure
3. Water Desalination
4. Water Filtration and Treatment
5. The Internet of Things (IoT)
6. A combination of all through a mutual fund or an ETF (exchange traded fund)

We will discuss companies that are in these segments, although we don't endorse any and are not investment advisors. These are presented as samples and examples of companies that operate within these segments and may nor may not capitalize on all of the potential opportunities that may arise.

In addition, you should consider the specific categories that have been identified by Citigroup as what it sees as the ten trends in the water industry:

1. Desalination systems
2. Water reuse technologies
3. Produced water / water utilities
4. Membranes for filtration
5. Ultraviolet (UV) disinfection

6. Ballast-water treatment technologies
7. Forward osmosis used in desalination
8. Water-efficiency technologies and products
9. Point-of-use treatment systems
10. Chinese competitors in water

Keep in mind that while we discuss these areas, Michael Burry has, as usual, taken a different path in his quest to invest in what he sees as the greatest water opportunity.

Dr. Burry, a physician and hedge fund manager, believes that the most efficient way to invest in water is through agriculture. He believes that transporting water is impractical and so the purchase of water rights makes no sense to him. Instead, he thinks that if you grow food in water rich areas and transport it for sale to water poor areas, it is the best way to redistribute water, and should be the most profitable. Consequently, much of his water investing has been through the purchase of farmland.

This may sound crazy to some people, but we have all learned that Dr. Burry has a knack for understanding and spotting unexpected events that very few other people have predicted, if any.

The one thing about Dr. Burry that you should remember is that he believes predicting economic events is possible if you do enough background work to fully understand what is happening. With the housing crisis, he is one of the only people who read almost every prospectus written for the toxic mortgage bonds that were being sold, which amounts to hundreds of pages for each one, in very fine print, and written in thick legalese. To him the failure of the mortgage market was inevitable, because he understood and knew what was really being sold to investors, even when the brokers, investors, regulators, rating companies, and others completely ignored the warning signs. Maybe grandpa's farm was a pretty good idea after all.

Now let's take the segments of the water industry that we have identified, and talk about some of the companies in those segments. Of course, some of them will overlap in segments, but we will try to discuss them in some logical order. Keep in mind that we do not recommend any of these companies, but we use them here as an illustration of the types of companies in these segments that you should begin to investigate for possible investment. Remember that there are over 400 water-related companies in the world, so your homework is cut out for you!

Water Utilities

American Water (NYSE: AWK), the largest publicly traded water company in the world, not only has its own set of treated water storage facilities, but offers services to both residential and business areas in pipeline repair and upkeep. The company has 49,000 miles of water mains and collection pipes, and offers its repair services to 47 states and customers in Ontario, Canada.

As of September 2016, the company had closed 10 acquisitions in six states that brought in more than 1,500 new water customers and about 6,000 new wastewater customers. Another 16 such acquisitions in eight states aims to bring in more than 70,000 customers later in the year.

American Water has had consistent dividend raises. Since 2012, the payout has had a CAGR of 11%, and has equaled between 50% and 60% of the company's net income.

The second largest water utility is Aqua America (NYSE: AWK), which is a company that has made 300 acquisitions over the past two decades. The company serves approximately 3 million people in Pennsylvania, Ohio, North Carolina, Illinois, Texas, New Jersey, Indiana and Virginia. The company was founded in 1886 as the Springfield Water Company. Aqua America grew by acquisition, but it was not until the early 1990s that it really began to buy up as many water related companies as it could find, and became the behemoth that it is today. As we write this, the stock is in the $30/share range.

United Utilities Group PLC is a public limited company, with a primary listing of its shares on the London Stock Exchange. The company was formed after water utilities were permitted to be privately owned in the United Kingdom in 1989. United Utilities holds a license to provide water and sewage services to around seven million people in North West England. These services are regulated with the water regulator, Ofwat, which reviews the company's price limits every five years. Between 2010 and 2015, the company invested more than £3 billion to improve the water and wastewater infrastructure and the environment across North West England, covering: over 42,000 kilometers of water pipes, from Cumbria to Cheshire; over 76,000 kilometers of sewers; 569 wastewater treatment works; 94 water treatment works; over 56,000 hectares of catchment land.

Infrastructure

As mentioned above, there is an overlap in these segments, and both American Water and Aqua America are constantly improving the infrastructure of the subsidiaries that they acquire, so look at them from the infrastructure position also. For example, Aqua America operates regulated utilities that provide water or wastewater services in the United States. Specifically, this company offers these services through operating and maintenance contracts with municipal authorities and other parties.

Furthermore, Aqua America also provides water and wastewater line repair services and protection solutions to households; inspects, cleans, and repairs storm and sanitary wastewater lines; installs and tests devices that prevent the contamination of potable water; designs and builds water and wastewater systems; and offers non-utility raw water supply services for firms in the natural gas drilling industry.

Aqua America owns and operates more than 1,400 water systems and 187 wastewater treatment plants and collection systems. The company's infrastructure footprint as of the end of 2015 includes over 12,500 miles of water main, 20 surface water filtration plants, 183 wastewater treatment plants, in excess of 3,000 wells, over 860 water storage tanks, and more than 1,100 vehicles (some of which are powered by CNG).

While some companies have been struggling to maintain dividend payouts or outright cutting them, Aqua America's dividend is in no danger of either. To gauge the stability of a company's dividend, we typically look to its payout ratio (a company's payout ratio is simply the proportion of earnings it pays out as dividends). In other words, the lower a payout ratio percentage is, the better and more secure its dividends are. Between 2010 and 2013, Aqua America managed to lower its payout ratio from nearly 75% to around 53%. In 2015, it was roughly 55%.

Additional companies that we noticed in the infrastructure segment include the following:

Calgon Carbon (CCC) is a manufacturer of products that remove contaminants and odors from liquids and gases, for industrial, municipal, and consumer markets. Calgon has a somewhat interesting and different niche. The company offers carbon technologies used in over 700 distinct market applications from purifying air and drinking water, to purifying foods and pharmaceuticals, to separating gas and removing mercury emissions from coal-powered electrical facilities. The company touts itself as a leader in the activated carbon industry. With ultraviolet light disinfection and oxidation expertise, Calgon has originated purification systems for drinking water, wastewater, odor control, pollution abatement, and a variety of industrial and commercial manufacturing processes.

Mueller Water Products (NYSE: MWA) is one of the largest manufacturers and distributors of fire hydrants, pipe fittings, and valves in North America. The company is a manufacturer and marketer of products and services used in the transmission, distribution and measurement of water in North America. Its product and service portfolio includes engineered valves, fire hydrants, metering products and systems, leak detection, and pipe condition assessment. The company assists municipalities to operational efficiencies, improve customer service and prioritize capital spending.

Xylem (NYSE: XYL) is a manufacturer of pumps, valves and analytic equipment used to move, test, and treat water in more than 150 countries. In 2011, Xylem completed its spinoff from ITT Corporation. The company owns subsidiaries serving clean water delivery, wastewater transport and treatment, dewatering, and analytical instrumentation.

Pentair PLC (NYSE: PNR) is a multinational diversified industrial company incorporated in Ireland with tax residency in UK, with its main U.S. office located in Minneapolis, Minnesota. As of 2015, half of its revenue was derived from the United States. With fiscal year 2015 revenues of US$6.43 billion, Pentair employs more than 30,000 people worldwide. The company has grown primarily by acquisition. In August 1999, Pentair bought the DeVilbiss Air Power Company. DeVilbiss makes air compressors, pressure washers, and generators, which complemented Pentair's professional Pneumatics tools that were powered by air compressors such as DeWalt and Porter-Cable.

In 2004, Pentair bought WICOR Industries, the former water systems subsidiary of Wisconsin Energy. WICOR made water pumps, filters, and pool equipment components under the Sta-Rite, SHURflo, and Hypro brands. In 2006, Pentair purchased Germany-based Jung Pumpen GmbH, which makes pumps and other products for wastewater processing.

Water Desalination

France is the heavy hitter when it comes to desalination plant building and operation, even though the United States and Saudi Arabia have the most desalination plants in the world.

Veolia (OTC: VEOEY) is a French company with businesses in water, environmental services, and energy services and transportation. It has over 1,700 desalination plants in more than 80 countries.

Veolia extended its contract with the Milwaukee Metropolitan Sewerage District for its ongoing wastewater collection and treatment services. The company's business is to provide clean water to customers and collect wastewater to either be safely discharged or recycled.

This is where the treatments come in: Veolia uses both biological and membrane technologies to decontaminate water. It has a particular interest in providing and recycling the water used in shale fracking, a water-intensive industry. This contract amounts to $500 million in income for the company.

Veolia also offers an annual dividend which stands at 3.7% per share.

The U.S. company General Electric (NYSE: GE) also has a large, global stake in water desalination. It operates the largest desalination plant in Africa: located in Algiers, the Hamma plant supplies the city with 53 million gallons of drinking water per day. GE also powers one of the world's largest desalination plants in Australia and the largest wastewater treatment facility in the world in Abu Dhabi.

In April 2015, GE also began installing its own bioreactor membranes into Stockholm's Henriksdal water treatment plant. These membranes are made of a special synthetic resin and undulate to clean the water faster, better, and at a much lower price.

GE's reach into several sectors gives it the freedom to expand its different technologies. Even when the company isn't operating its own plants, it is powering and improving upon others. Its steady dividend payout of $0.23 per share shows it also has plenty to spare for its supporters.

Water Filtration and Treatment

Once again, remember that both Veolia and GE also fit into this category.

Dow Chemical Co. (NYSE: DOW) water division is a major player in the water treatment game. It won an innovation award for its Tequatic Plus filter, which treats high-solids water. The company reduces the energy needed to treat water efficiently and has expanded the world's wastewater reuse options. Its Filmtec Eco reverse osmosis technology in 2014 provided 40% better water purification ability using 30% less energy than previous technologies.

Dow also has holdings in Saudi Arabia, where it's contracted the Sadara Chemical Company to construct a membrane fabrication facility. It has also launched a large-scale pilot project at the King Abdullah University of Science and Technology to access seawater from the Red Sea and use it to experiment with new purification technologies on an industrial scale.

And keeping up well with our lineup of water treatment companies, Dow's dividend rose from $0.42 in early 2015 to $0.46 per diluted share in 2016.

The Internet of Things (IoT)

By now, most people have heard that the next "big thing" is the Internet of Things. The Internet of Things is the ongoing trend of items (your phone, your watch, your glasses, your car, your coffee pot, your pet feeder) being connected to the internet or the cloud. Many industries are using this technology to monitor their systems and increase productivity and efficiency.

Water is no different. Watertech Capital's Stephen Hoffman says the niche of the Internet of Things as it relates to water will grow 14 to 16% annually for the next several years. As with everything, the future of water is becoming computerized, digitized, analyzed, and connected to the internet.

Badger Meter Inc. (NYSE: BMI) is a U.S. company with a wide reach. It sells mechanical and electronic water meters and products to measure and control goods that travel via pipes. These include water, wastewater, oil, and gas, among other things.

Badger's meters monitor water usage so customers can be aware of what they're using and what the utilities are charging them for. The utilities use them for billing as well. 75% of the company's meter sales go to municipal water systems.

In January 2014, the company introduced a new product, the BEACON Advanced Metering Analytics system, which provides a cellular residential radio and allows customers the ability to download an app (EyeOnWater) to monitor their water usage any time on any mobile device. Since then, the company has extended its advanced metering analytics offerings with additional devices compatible with the BEACON meter.

Badger acquired its largest distributor, National Meter and Automation Inc., in October 2014. This provided the company not only with stronger control over its distribution, but services for its customers including meter testing and installation, water audits, and leak detection.

In 2016, the company's services were deemed strong enough to be awarded a contract with American Water. As the utility grows its customer base, this company and its devices are reaping the rewards.

Itron Inc. (NYSE: ITRI) offers similar meters for electricity, gas, and water. Its meters also measure use of water for both residential and business use. And, like Badger, the information is available through software, so customers can always be aware of the data being collected.

Itron, however, goes a step further in offering data interpretation as a service. First, it has analysis software available to customers which uses the collected data to make short- and long-term predictions about the customer's water use and costs. It also has a subsidiary called Private Cloud which allows businesses to save their usage information and consult with Itron experts to come up with efficiency solutions, and those experts are available for consultations for all customers. Its Professional Services include installation services, system maintenance and training, and technical support.

Where Badger has more ease of use, Itron is built for in-depth information processing. Both use Internet of Things technology to make saving water easier.

The IoT market at large is growing exponentially as data collection and analysis become the key to operational efficiency. Nowhere is this development more necessary than in today's drought-stricken water market.

A combination of all through a mutual fund or an ETF (exchange traded fund)

Guggenheim S&P Global Water Index ETF (the Fund), formerly Claymore S&P Global Water Index ETF seeks investment results that correspond generally to the performance of an equity index called the S&P Global Water NR Index. The S&P Global Water NR Index consists of approximately 50 equity securities selected based on investment and other criteria, from a universe of companies listed on global developed market exchanges.

The Index is designed to have a balanced representation from different segments of the water industry consisting of two clusters: 25 water utilities and infrastructure companies and 25 water equipment and materials companies based upon Standard & Poor's Capital IQ industry classification. The Fund will invest at least 90% of its total assets in common stock and American depository receipts that comprise the Index depository receipts representing common stocks included in the Index. The Fund's investment advisor is Guggenheim Funds Investment Advisors, LLC.

To invest directly in the commercialization of proven AWG patented technology and research, the premier company appears to be World Environmental Solutions (WES). The company is headed by Walter Ivison as the CEO of both the Australian entity WES and the JV company MultiChill Technologies Inc. in Toledo, Ohio.

Summary

Is our interest as investors in water, its cleanliness or its scarcity? Do we invest in the bottlers, rebuilders of the infrastructure, utility consolidators, filter companies, or perhaps desalination? Interesting choices. Our personal futures and fortunes depend on a steady supply of clean drinking water. Will we eventually trade water futures? Or is that already a reality?

EPILOGUE – ENERGY

Water is an enigma in that it is ubiquitous and yet scarce. While it is everywhere, in many parts of the world it exists in a form that is not fit for human consumption. The focus of this book has been the problems and potential solutions relating to access to water that is safe for humans, so that we can sustain life (known in the trade as "potable water").

There is a theme that underlies and runs throughout all of the chapters of this book. That theme, always lurking in the background, is the part that energy plays in the big picture of potable water.

To obtain potable water, and to get it to the human user, it is inevitable that energy must be expended to obtain the end result. Therein lies the problem, particularly in the third world, where the expense of energy to reach this goal puts the poorest nations in the most jeopardy.

It has been said many times by non-U.S. people that Americans are so rich that they urinate into clean water. During the lifetime of all Americans, that has clearly been the case, and has never even occurred to us as Americans. For many foreigners, however, it is a blatant truth that they have difficulty in understanding. How could we be so careless with such a precious product?

Occasionally, Americans get a glimpse of a third world life, when problems like a Flint, Michigan disaster occur, or in the aftermath of a Hurricane Katrina where thousands are stranded without clean water for days on end. These problems appear on the news for a few days, and then are quickly forgotten by the American masses as more timely news occurs. To

Americans, these problems seem temporary and in their minds are quickly resolved. That is not the case in the third world, and may not be the case in America in the future.

One of the major trends that could make the entire situation worse is the growing population. According to the United Nations in 2015, the projections for world population go from 7.3 billion in 2015 to 8.5 billion in 2030, and 9.7 billion in 2050. The UN indicates that most of the population growth will take place in nine high fertility countries, most of which are in Africa. The population of Nigeria is anticipated to exceed the population of the United States by 2050, making it the third largest country by population. Many of the countries where the highest population growth is taking place are presently struggling to deal with widespread poverty, and the consequent lack of clean water.

In Chapter 2 we discussed the bottled water industry, which lends itself to developed economies with citizens who can afford to pay the high cost associated with acquiring bottled water for personal consumption on a regular basis. Is the cost of this a viable option for the entire world for the future? Without being able to obtain clean water on a continuing basis at a reasonable price, will the stability of Africa and other high growth, but low income areas and nations, succumb to water war chaos, or fall victim to the influence of radical groups like ISIS? Can we find a cheap enough power source to solve this problem to avoid more volatility in the world?

In Chapter 3 we described how the United States needs a complete renovation of our entire water infrastructure, which will be very energy consuming and consequently expensive. This effort in the United States will put a strain on our resources to accomplish a massive task created by letting our infrastructure deteriorate over many years. Projects like this will be needed also in the third world, and will require large amounts of inexpensive energy to accomplish. Just as cheap oil built America, a cheap energy source will be needed to bring clean water to the third world.

In Chapter 4 we focused on all of the toxic chemicals in our water and the potential negative effect of those chemicals. What is needed to remove those chemicals from our water? Energy, and lots of it. What is the cost of that energy?

Chapter 5 related to the oil and gas industry and the prevalence of fracking today. Many people believe that the fracking process threatens our aquifers and puts us in jeopardy of having a serious water crisis in America. Fracking benefits America by reducing our dependence on foreign oil, yet puts us in potential jeopardy of poisoning our water. In this case, the production of energy possibly works against our need to provide clean water for our citizens. In countries like Nigeria, which is oil rich, fracking may also contribute to the risk of unacceptable water quality.

Chapters 6 and 7 described the risks related to lead, fluoride, and other additives or contaminants to clean water. Removal of these substances can be accomplished; it just takes the use of an energy source.

The additional chapters reviewed water treatment and filtration as well as removing water from the atmosphere as one potential solution to obtaining potable water. What all of these things have in common is that they need an energy source to either pump the water through filters, inject the water with various treatments or pull the moisture (water) from the air. In the case of the water from air concept, the amount of energy needed is directly proportional to the amount of moisture in the air, thus: less moisture, more energy.

This situation can be described in many ways, such as trading watts for water, or energy expended equals clean water. How will the goal of clean water for the planet be reached? How can be produce energy at an inexpensive enough level to solve these problems worldwide?

One approach is through the prize concept or challenge. Most of us don't know or remember that, when Lindberg completed the first transatlantic flight by himself, it was in response to a competition, or a reward challenge, called the Orteig Prize. The Orteig Prize was a reward offered to the first Allied aviator to fly non-stop from New York City to Paris or vice versa. The prize offered was $25,000, or about $350,000 in today's dollars.

But the prize money was not what most aviators and aircraft companies were seeking. They were seeking the prestige, advertising, and glory of accomplishing a task that many thought to be unobtainable. The result of this challenge and the advances in aviation were the result of many participants competing to win the challenge.

Similarly, the Ansari X Prize of $10,000,000, offered by the X Prize Foundation, was a competition for the first non-government organization to "build and launch a spacecraft capable of carrying three people to 100 kilometers above the Earth's surface, twice within two weeks." The prize was announced in 1996 as an incentive for the creation of inexpensive spaceflight. It was won in 2004 by Burt Rutan, and financed by Paul Allen, one of the Microsoft founders. It is believed that over $100 million was invested in new technologies by those vying for the $10 million prize.

Right now the X Prize Foundation and a related entity, HeroX, have a number of prize categories relating to water. Will this open source approach find the answer to clean, affordable water, through cheap energy? We have learned to never underestimate the creativity of the human mind.

www.ingramcontent.com/pod-product-compliance
Lightning Source LLC
Chambersburg PA
CBHW072123280526

45788CB00002B/518